PROPERTY

OF

GENERAL

SURGERY

*Atlas of Techniques in*

# BREAST SURGERY

# Atlas of Techniques in

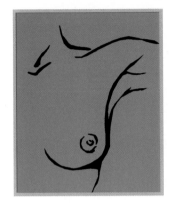

# BREAST SURGERY

**William Silen, MD, FACS**
Professor of Surgery
Harvard Medical School
Beth Israel Hospital
Boston, Massachusetts

**W. Earle Matory, Jr., MD, FACS**
Associate Professor
Division of Plastic and Reconstructive Surgery
University of Massachusetts Medical Center
Worcester, Massachusetts

**Susan M. Love, MD, FACS**
Director, UCLA Breast Center
Associate Professor of Clinical Surgery
University of California Los Angeles Medical School
Los Angeles, California

*Illustrations by William Winn*

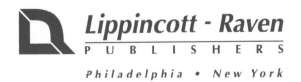

*Lippincott - Raven*
PUBLISHERS
*Philadelphia • New York*

*Acquisitions Editor:* Lisa McAllister
*Sponsoring Editor:* Emilie Linkins
*Project Editor:* Bridget Hannon Meyer
*Production Manager:* Caren Erlichman
*Senior Production Coordinator:* Kevin P. Johnson
*Designer:* Doug Smock
*Cover Designer:* Richard Merchán
*Indexer:* Ann Blum
*Compositor:* Tapsco, Incorporated
*Printer/Binder:* Quebecor/Kingsport
*Color Separator:* Jay's Publishers Services, Inc.

*Illustrations by William Winn*

**Library of Congress Cataloging-in-Publication Data**

Silen, William, 1927–
    Atlas of techniques in breast surgery/William Silen, W. Earle
Matory, Jr., Susan M. Love; illustrated by William Winn
        p. cm.
    Includes bibliographical references and index.
    ISBN 0-397-50946-4 (alk. paper)
    1. Breast—Cancer—Surgery—Atlases.    2. Breast—Surgery—Atlases.
I. Matory, W. Earle (William Earle), 1950–  .  II. Love, Susan M.
III. Title.
    [DNLM:  1. Breast Diseases—surgery—atlases.   2. Mastectomy—
methods—atlases.    3. Breast Neoplasms—surgery—atlases.
4. Mammaplasty—methods—atlases.   5. Breast—surgery—atlases.   WP
17 S582a 1996]
RD667.5.S55   1996
618.1′9059—dc20
DNLM/DLC
for Library of Congress                                                    95-19866
                                                                               CIP

9  8  7  6  5  4  3  2  1

## DEDICATION

To Ruth, whose patience, support and love have been my guiding lights.

Wᴏᴛʟʟɪᴀᴍ Sɪʟᴇɴ

To my father, William Earle Matory, Sr., ᴍᴅ, ꜰᴀᴄs, who has contributed so much to my life and that of so many others in so many ways.

W. Eᴀʀʟᴇ Mᴀᴛᴏʀʏ, Jʀ.

This book is dedicated to all of the women I have cared for over the years whose courage continues to push me to find better ways of treating breast disease.

Sᴜsᴀɴ M. Lᴏᴠᴇ

# Preface

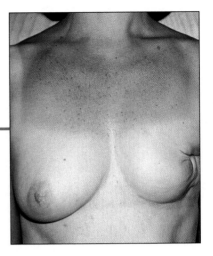

Recent changes in the diagnosis and treatment of diseases of the breast have resulted in the evolutionary development of a large number of new techniques, many of which were not part of the repertoire of the general surgeon of 25 or 30 years ago. For example, the problem of localization of the nonpalpable mammographically detected lesion simply did not exist because mammography was but a curiosity at that time. The recognition that local excision, combined with radiotherapy, is as effective as radical mastectomy for the treatment of invasive carcinoma has had a profound effect on the surgical techniques which are used to achieve local eradication of the lesion. Finally, the demonstration that immediate or delayed reconstruction of the breast does not adversely affect the outcome, as once thought, has led to widespread use of a variety of procedures to reconstruct the breast after treatment of the cancer.

While many of the newer techniques are regarded as being simple and uncomplicated, and are thus often relegated to a very junior person, the authors of this atlas have all too frequently observed deforming and untoward outcomes of local excisions of microcalcifications or partial mastectomies for carcinoma. We have been impressed that even surgeons of considerable experience are unaware of many of the principles which are requisite for an excellent cosmetic and functional result. Surprisingly, the literature on this subject has often been misleading and misguided. The procedures described in this atlas have been developed with plastic surgical principles in mind and have stood the test of time in the long-term clinical experience of the authors. Not only are appropriate procedures described in detail, but pitfalls to be avoided are also emphasized.

The atlas has been written for the audience of the general surgical practitioner, the surgical trainee, and for any student of surgery.

William Silen
W. Earle Matory, Jr.
Susan M. Love

# Foreword

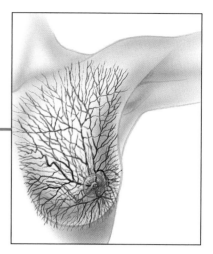

One of the major challenges confronting clinicians today is providing optimum treatment to patients with benign and malignant breast problems. Since surgical therapy is commonly used for these conditions, it is fitting that there should be up-to-date information outlining the techniques, principles and rationale for surgical treatment. This cogently written and well-illustrated book by Drs. Silen, Matory, and Love meets these goals in an admirable fashion. These authors meld their expertise in a highly informative way to answer commonly asked questions. They present an atlas of breast surgery emphasizing strategies which incorporate current diagnostic and therapeutic options.

Divided into five sections, the book encompasses the salient features of breast disease treatment in a logical way. Beginning with a discussion of applied anatomy and physiology, the authors outline basic concepts in the preservation of breast aesthetics. Particularly interesting is the emphasis on the use of resting skin tension lines, rather than Langer's lines, in the placement of incisions for various breast operations to ensure optimal cosmetic results. There follows a thorough discussion of the best methods to diagnose palpable and non-palpable lesions. The final section is concerned with surgical approaches for benign conditions, including the often troublesome recurrent periareolar abscess. The schematic diagrams used throughout the book are most helpful because they depict the various procedures in a clear and distinct manner. Appropriate description of operations for malignant neoplasms, ranging from partial to classical radical mastectomy, is presented.

There is an excellent section on post-mastectomy reconstruction including types of reconstruction and controversies in this area. Because of the greatly reduced use of silicone implants, the section on prosthetic devices has much less applicability. The discussion on use of autologous tissues and nipple–areolar reconstruction is well done and has increasing clinical use.

This book meets its goals and objectives and has done so in a highly effective manner. Clinicians who manage patients with breast diseases will be well served by the principles espoused here. The three authors—all recognized experts in the field— have produced an excellent book from which patients will benefit immeasurably. And for physicians and surgeons, patients always assume the role of primacy.

LaSalle Leffall, MD

# Contents

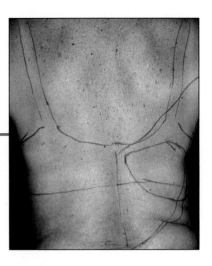

*Atlas of Techniques in*
# BREAST SURGERY

*Atlas of Techniques in Breast Surgery,*
by William Silen, W. Earle Matory, Jr. and Susan M. Love.
Lippincott-Raven Publishers, Philadelphia, © 1996.

# Introduction

A s long ago as the eighteenth century, the serious and life-threatening characteristics of carcinoma of the breast were an important driving force for surgeons to attempt aggressive surgical ablation of this disease.

Twenty-five years ago, there were few options in the treatment of breast cancer. The initial complaint was invariably that of a palpable mass. The patient was admitted to the hospital the night before surgery, knowing that on the following day a biopsy would be performed under general anesthesia. If a frozen section showed a carcinoma, the patient was subjected to a radical mastectomy without being awakened to be informed of the pathologic findings.

An atlas of breast surgery would have included one operation, radical mastectomy (Fig. I-1*A*). The necessity for this book reflects the changing times. A new paradigm of breast cancer has evolved and therefore the surgical approach must change with it. We now concede that many or most breast cancers have already metastasized by the time of initial diagnosis. The focus of physicians caring for patients having breast cancer has shifted from local to systemic control. Axillary lymph node dissection is now performed as much for its value in prognosis as for its value in prevention of regional recurrence. Local control can be achieved using less mutilating procedures than total, modified, or radical mastectomy (Fig. I-2, *left* and *right*). These advances in our understanding of the biology of breast cancer have significantly altered the philosophy of current therapeutic approaches.

Diagnostic procedures on the breast in the past were so frequently followed by mastectomy that little attention was given to the technique of "minor" operations, such as incisional or excisional biopsies. Local excisions were usually relegated to the most junior members of the surgical team, needle biopsy was thought to be inadequate and potentially harmful, and mammograms were not available. Excision of all breast masses was considered to be the only acceptable diagnostic maneuver. Many women with mul-

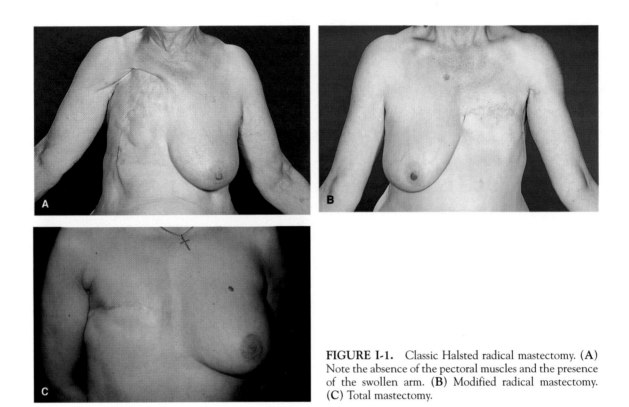

**FIGURE I-1.** Classic Halsted radical mastectomy. **(A)** Note the absence of the pectoral muscles and the presence of the swollen arm. **(B)** Modified radical mastectomy. **(C)** Total mastectomy.

tiple benign cysts were disfigured by repeated operations that failed to consider the cosmetic outcome. To some extent, these rigid "principles," often lacking scientific foundation, continue to influence current practice. New diagnostic techniques such as fine-needle aspiration, wire localizations, and stereotactic core-needle biopsies have significantly altered the approach to the patient with a breast mass.

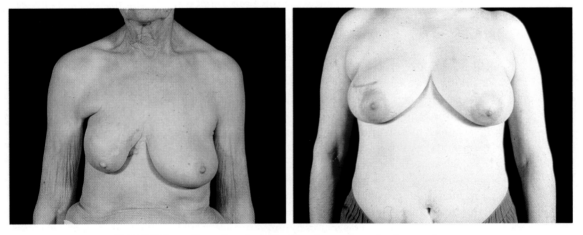

**FIGURE I-2.** Examples of results of local excision and radiation therapy.

Breast conservation for the treatment of mammary cancer has brought aesthetics into the realm of the surgeon. All operative procedures on the breast have the potential to result in loss of symmetry, alteration of the natural conical shape of the breast, and change in nipple position. Individuals who wish to avoid mastectomy are seeking removal of the cancer with minimal disfigurement. One must understand that the surgeon and oncologist compare the deformity of partial mastectomy with the appearance of the opposite normal breast, whereas the patient compares what may be a deformed breast to the alternative of no breast at all. Biopsies and partial mastectomies must therefore incorporate these considerations. Even the tried and true mastectomy must be altered if reconstruction is to follow. For example, the trend toward the preservation of breast skin simplifies reconstructive alternatives and inherently improves the aesthetic outcome.

Current approaches in addressing breast cancer must include the goals of ablation of the malignancy, cosmesis, and preservation of sensibility. The combined expertise of the breast surgeon and the plastic surgeon is indispensable. An attempt is made herein to reconcile the diverse goals of breast conservation, cosmesis, and eradication of malignancy and to present a scientifically founded and practical approach to the management of breast disease.

# *Part* I

# Anatomic and Cosmetic Considerations in Breast Surgery

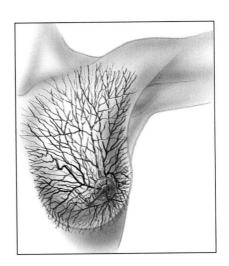

*Atlas of Techniques in Breast Surgery,*
by William Silen, W. Earle Matory, Jr. and Susan M. Love.
Lippincott-Raven Publishers, Philadelphia, © 1996.

# *Chapter* 1

# Applied Anatomy and Physiology

Anatomic architecture and physiologic principles guide diagnostic and therapeutic approaches to managing any organ system. Applied anatomic, physiologic, and plastic surgical concepts are presented as a basis for the surgeon's management of breast disease in the next decade.

## ✦ *EMBRYOLOGY*

During the sixth week of intrauterine life, the cutaneous epithelium of the pectoral region in the embryo differentiates, forming mammary buds (Fig. 1-1). These buds develop along a milk ridge that usually extends from the axilla to the groin. Although supernumerary breasts can persist in the adult anywhere along the milk line, the nipple–areolar complex develops primarily at the level of the fourth intercostal space. Before the onset of puberty in both sexes, a breast bud is palpable beneath the areola. During puberty, estrogen induces development into a hemispheric and subsequently conical breast structure. Temporary or permanent asymmetric development may occur in either gender during pubescence, usually as a result of variable end-organ response. Pubescent males may develop gynecomastia, possibly due to abnormal estrogen–testosterone ratios.[1] Asymmetry in the male and female are common during this stage of development and also in adults. Differences in the size of the breasts usually stabilize within 1 to 2 years of the onset of puberty. Therefore, it is preferable to wait for the completion of secondary sexual changes before addressing gynecomastia or asymmetry surgically if such is deemed appropriate. Gynecomastia, when present in the later stages of sexual development, is usually permanent and amenable to surgical reduction.

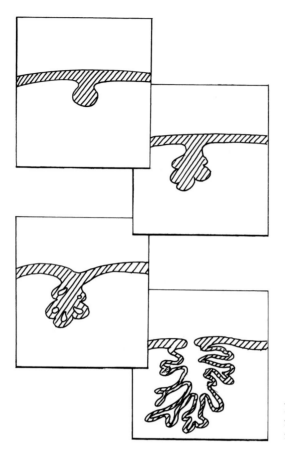

**FIGURE 1-1.** The mammary bud arises from the cutaneous epithelium of the milk ridge.

## ✦ *NORMAL BREAST*

The normal external breast extends from the second rib to the sixth or seventh rib, where the inframammary fold is located (Fig. 1-2). Mammary tissue extends from the mid-axillary line at the edge of the latissimus dorsi medially to the lateral sternal border.[2] About 5% of breast tissue is found in other areas.[2] Breast parenchyma has been identified at the level of the clavicle, across the mid-sternum, and along the upper abdominal wall superficial to the anterior rectus fascia (Fig. 1-3A).[3] In addition, an axillary projection of the breast, forming the tail, may extend as far laterally as the posterior axillary line (see Fig. 1-3B). Thus, the dissection for total mastectomy should extend from the level of the clavicle to the superior portion of the rectus fascia and from the mid-sternum to the edge of the latissimus.

During adolescence, the breast is hemispheric, with the nipple–areolar complex located at the fourth intercostal interspace. With maturation, the upper breast becomes less convex and more flattened (Fig. 1-4). As the breast enlarges, the lower pole becomes more full. The nipple is normally located at or just above the level of the inframammary fold. Aging, postpartum involution, and weight loss may all contribute to laxity of the skin and supporting ligaments of the breast. As aging and gravitational forces progress, a redistribution of breast parenchyma and skin results in a lower nipple position or nipple ptosis. Sagging of breast parenchyma below the inframammary fold is called pseudoptosis.

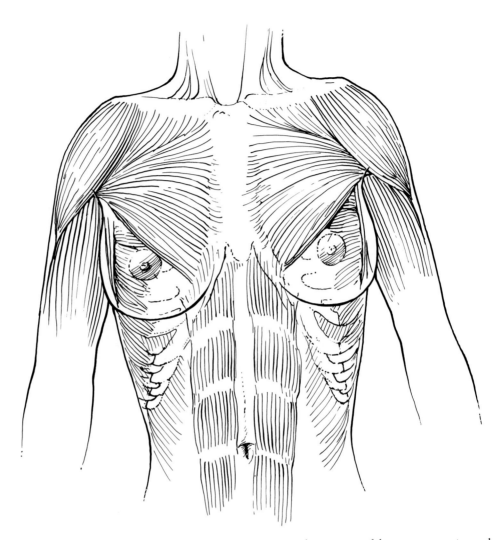

**FIGURE 1-2.**  The breast covers the pectoralis major muscle, a portion of the serratus anterior, and some of the rectus sheath and costal cartilages.

## Fascia

The breast is a skin appendage encapsulated within superficial and deep layers of the superficial fascia (Fig. 1-5). A layer of loose areolar tissue usually separates breast parenchyma from the pectoral fascia. Superiorly, the lower fibers of the platysma distinctly course between the superficial and deep layers of the superficial fascia.[4] Elsewhere, the deep layer of the superficial fascia and the superficial layer of the pectoral fascia are clinically indistinct. The pectoral fascia covers the pectoralis major and is contiguous with the deep fascia of the rectus abdominis, serratus anterior, and external oblique muscles. Laterally, the superficial and deep pectoral fascia merge to form a sheath that envelops the axillary vessels. This envelope contains sizable lymphatic cords and axillary lymph nodes, which are routinely excised during axillary dissection.

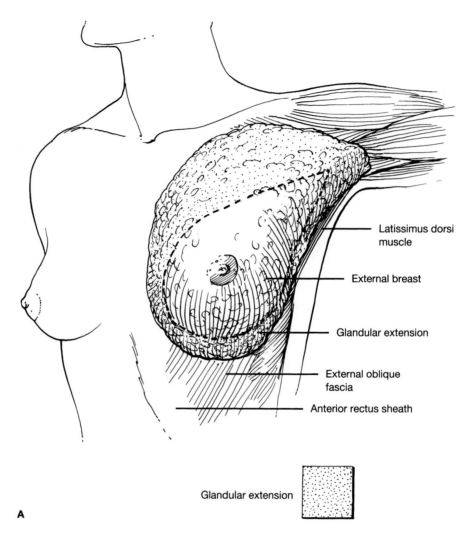

Latissimus dorsi muscle

External breast

Glandular extension

External oblique fascia

Anterior rectus sheath

Glandular extension

**A**

**FIGURE 1-3.**  (**A**) Breast parenchyma has been noted at the level of the clavicle, to the midline of the sternum, and in the upper abdominal wall along the superior rectus fascia. (**B**) An axillary projection of the breast, forming the tail of the breast, may extend as far laterally as the midaxillary line.

Cooper's suspensory ligaments course throughout the breast, interconnecting the dermis, the superficial and deep layers of the superficial fascia, and the pectoralis major muscle fascia (see Fig. 1-5). Stretching and lengthening of the suspensory ligaments as a result of aging, gravity, weight loss, and atrophy (e.g., after pregnancy) contribute to ptosis. Occasionally, projections of breast tissue extend into the dermis. This intimate relation of breast parenchyma and the dermis has been the rationale for elevation of thin skin flaps during mastectomy. Generally, however, the anterior layer of the superficial fascia encapsulates most breast tissue. When visible, this fascia serves as a guide to the surgeon in developing the plane of dissection between subcutaneous fat and glandular breast.

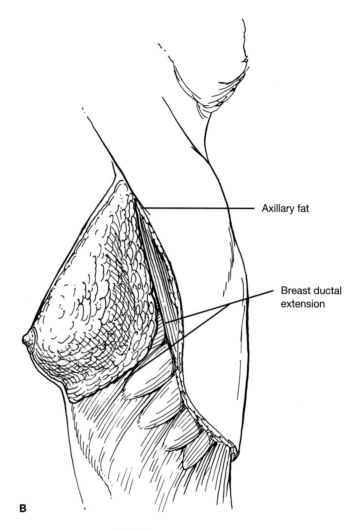

Axillary fat

Breast ductal
extension

B

**FIGURE 1-3.** *(Continued)*

## Glandular Architecture and Ductal Systems

Little attention has been paid to the anatomic arrangement of breast ducts. Cooper,[5] in 1840, injected soft wax of different colors into the ducts and showed that there are several separate ductal systems. The branches of these systems weave extensively and intertwine but do not communicate with each other (Fig. 1-6). Subsequently, Hicken[3] demonstrated the expansive ductal architecture by ductograms. Sartorius[5a] (personal communication with Susan Love) has performed numerous ductograms on women with normal and abnormal breasts. His work suggests that five to nine ducts have a fairly consistent pattern, with one duct lying directly posterior to the nipple, one extending medially, and another laterally at three and nine o'clock, respectively. Most variations in ductal pattern are in the superior and inferior breast, where each of these areas may have one, two, or three separate ductal systems. The main ducts are formed by the coalescence of many smaller branches.

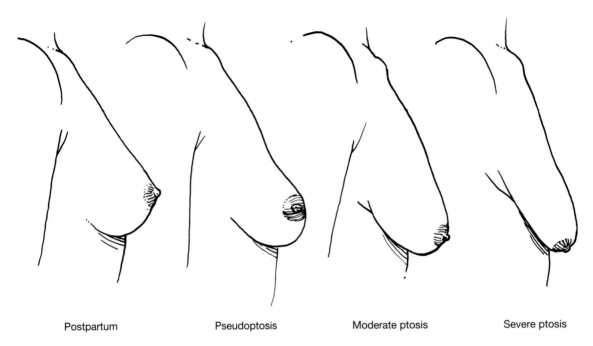

| Postpartum | Pseudoptosis | Moderate ptosis | Severe ptosis |

**FIGURE 1-4.** As aging proceeds, there is often a redistribution of breast parenchyma and skin causing a lower position of the nipple. This change is known as ptosis of the nipple. Dropping of the breast parenchyma below the inframammary fold is referred to as pseudoptosis.

Major ducts widen slightly into the lactiferous sinuses, which then pass through a spiral subnipple muscle and emerge through the nipple. In addition to the major ducts, which are connected to breast parenchyma, there are five to 10 blind openings in the nipple, which have no communication with the mammary parenchyma. These are thought to be sebaceous glands, which may help to provide lubrication for the nipple.

At the terminal end of each ductule is the lobule, which is responsible for secreting milk. Breast cancer is thought to start at the junction of the terminal duct and the lobule. Whether in situ carcinoma begins in one ductal–lobular unit and spreads along the duct or whether it arises simultaneously from many foci within one duct has yet to be determined. At least one study has shown ductal hyperplasia and ductal carcinoma in situ (DCIS) to be monoclonal,[5b] and anatomic studies confirm that DCIS is often found throughout a single ductal system.[5c]

Some have termed the duct with all of its branches and lobules, a "lobe." This terminology can be misleading because it implies that there are distinct, easily identifiable anatomically defined lobes analogous to those in the lung. The ducts of one major ductal system do not communicate with those of another but the branches of one system intertwine with those of others, making the anatomic designation of a lobe impossible. Multiple lobules, which are often widely dispersed, coalesce and drain into ductules that ultimately join to form a series of radially oriented ducts that surface at the nipple (see Fig. 1-6). Neoplastic proliferation along the length of a single duct may therefore appear to involve multiple areas of the breast. Traditional orientation of the breast biopsy or lumpectomy has been in the transverse di-

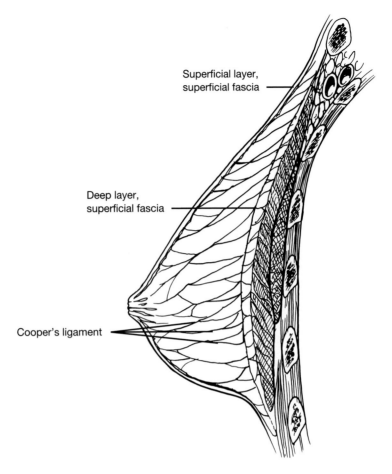

Superficial layer, superficial fascia

Deep layer, superficial fascia

Cooper's ligament

**FIGURE 1-5.** Cooper's ligaments course throughout the breast connecting the dermis, the superficial and deep layers of the superficial fascia, and the pectoralis major muscle fascia.

rection, often yielding only a cross-section of the radially oriented ductal system. Given the radial and lobular anatomic alignment of the ductal systems, a radially oriented parenchymal resection theoretically will yield a more accurate sampling of a ductal system (Fig. 1-7A).

The terms "quadrant" or "quadrantectomy" are often used to describe the location of a lesion or a type of resection. Although these terms describe a gross region of the breast, there is no specific ductal or lobular correlate. A tumor may be interpreted as being "multicentric" because of its location in multiple "quadrants" of the breast.[6] A more accurate interpretation would be that there is involvement of one ductal system that spans several regions of the breast. This was nicely demonstrated by Holland and coworkers, who observed that whereas DCIS may often be found in more than one gross quadrant of the breast, direct contiguity of DCIS could nevertheless be demonstrated in most cases.[6,7] This study suggests that DCIS is often confined to one ductal system. If a reliable anatomic map of the ductal system were available to the surgeon preoperatively, excisional biopsy might be accomplished in a more logical and consistent fashion.

*(text continues on p. 17)*

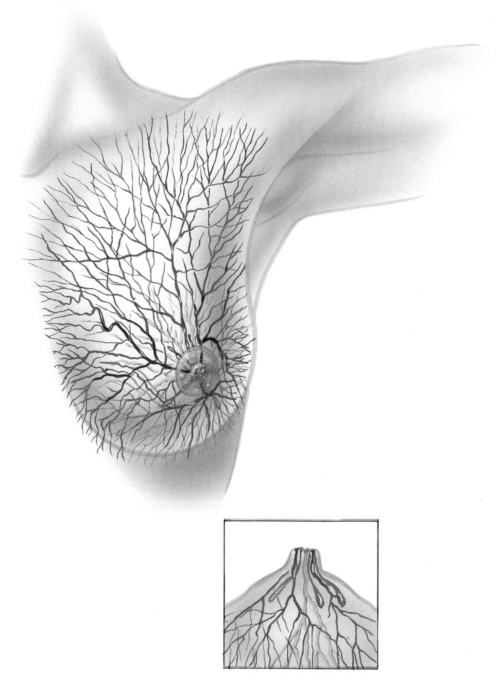

**FIGURE 1-6.** The ductal systems are radially oriented but intertwine and overlap. There is generally no communication between them. Five to nine ducts have a fairly consistent distribution. One lies directly posterior to the nipple, one is directed medially, and one laterally.

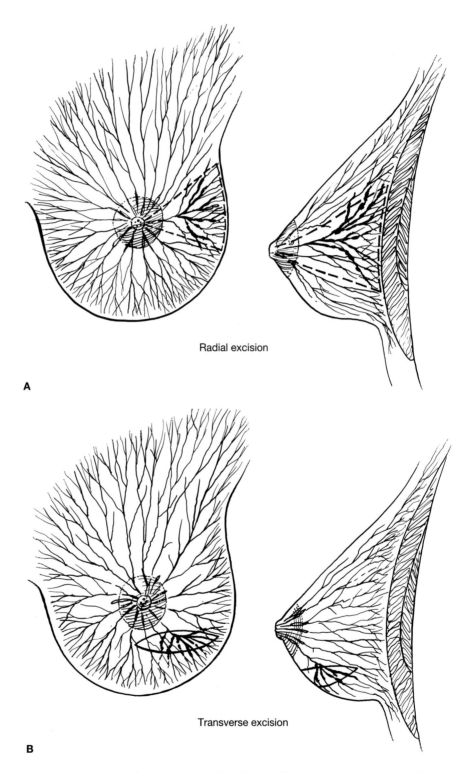

Radial excision

**A**

Transverse excision

**B**

**FIGURE 1-7.** **(A)** A radial excision depicted by the *dotted line* is more likely to excise a lesion that extends along the ductal system than **(B)** a transverse excision (*solid ellipse*).

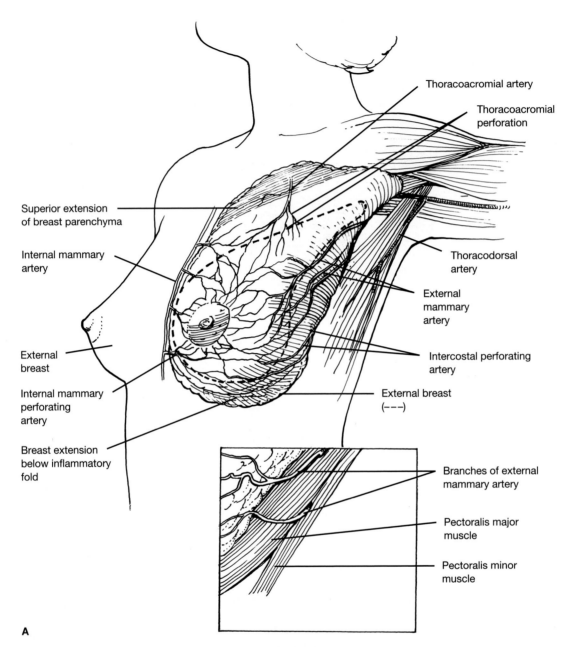

Thoracoacromial artery

Thoracoacromial perforation

Superior extension of breast parenchyma

Internal mammary artery

Thoracodorsal artery

External mammary artery

External breast

Intercostal perforating artery

Internal mammary perforating artery

External breast (–––)

Breast extension below inflammatory fold

Branches of external mammary artery

Pectoralis major muscle

Pectoralis minor muscle

**A**

**FIGURE 1-8.** (A) Four sources of arterial inflow: the thoracoacromial artery, internal mammary artery, external mammary (lateral thoracic), and the intercostal perforators. (B) The internal mammary and intercostal arteries provide branches that perforate the intercostal muscles.

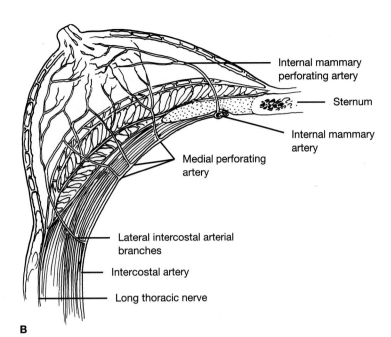

Internal mammary perforating artery

Sternum

Internal mammary artery

Medial perforating artery

Lateral intercostal arterial branches

Intercostal artery

Long thoracic nerve

B

**FIGURE 1-8.**  *(Continued)*

## Parenchyma

*Alpha streptococcus* and *Staphylococcus epidermitis* can be cultured from normal breast tissue. The presence of these organisms is thought to be because of the communication of the ductal system with the skin. Because of this indigenous bacterial flora, perioperative antibiotics may be appropriate, particularly when breast implants are used.

Fat is primarily responsible for the bulk and shape of the breast. The amount of fat varies considerably with the individual and with age. The fat-to-gland ratio increases after menopause, commensurate with glandular atrophy and weight gain. Adipose tissue within the postmenopausal breast has diminished blood supply, thus increasing the likelihood of fat necrosis after any manipulation of breast tissue, including surgery, radiation, trauma, or infection.

In the younger patient, subcutaneous fat is distinct from the superficial fascia and underlying breast. With aging and laxity of the fascia, the superficial border of the breast becomes less distinct as stromal and lobular atrophy progress. The subcutaneous fat and superficial fascia blend with each other, thus making identification of the subcutaneous–glandular plane more difficult.

## Arterial Supply

Four primary sources contribute to arterial inflow of the breast: the thoracoacromial artery, internal mammary artery, the intercostal perforators, and the lateral thoracic artery (Fig. 1-8*A*). The thoracoacromial artery, a major source of blood supply to the pectoralis major muscle, sends perforating branches

17

through the muscle that provide circulation to the overlying breast and skin. The internal mammary artery is an important source of blood flow to the pectoral muscles and also has branches that perforate the intercostal muscles along the lateral border of the sternum to supply the medial breast (see Fig. 1-8*B*). The second and third internal mammary perforators are usually the largest of the perforating vessels and supply the upper breast. The intercostal perforators of the second through sixth interspace supply the pectoralis major, breast, and skin. The fourth through sixth intercostal perforating vessels make a significant contribution to the central and lateral breast. The lateral thoracic, also known as the external mammary artery, is usually a direct branch of the axillary artery but may arise from the subscapular artery. This vessel serves as a primary source of blood to the lateral pectoralis major and minor and to the lateral upper breast.

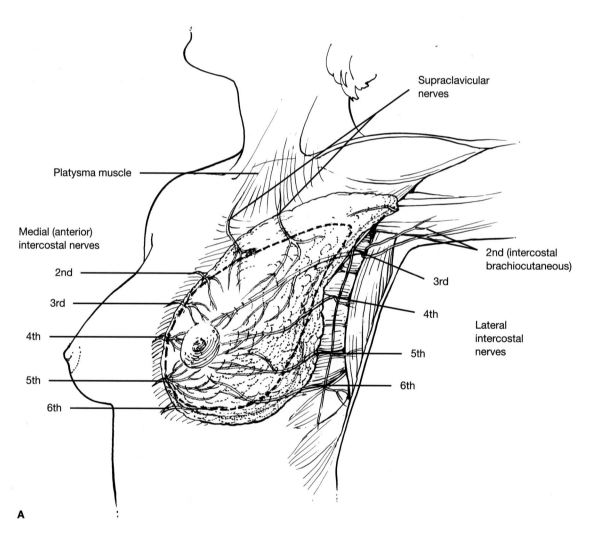

**FIGURE 1-9.** (**A** and **B**) The nerve supply to the breast arises from the third through sixth intercostal nerves.

### Venous Drainage

The venous drainage of the breast consists of superficial and deep venous plexuses.[4] The superficial plexus originates in the periareolar area and courses just anterior to the superficial fascia, with interconnections across the midline. Drainage is primarily upward and medially. The superficial and deep plexuses communicate by vessels passing through the breast parenchyma.

Deep venous drainage accompanies the arterial flow. Intercostal veins course through the azygos and vertebral veins to the superior vena cava. The internal thoracic perforators empty into the innominate vein. Pectoral perforators flow into the lateral thoracic vein, which ultimately reaches the axillary vein.

### Nerves

Sensory innervation arises from the third through sixth intercostal nerves (Fig. 1-9*A* and *B*). The second intercostal or the intercostal brachiocutaneous nerve courses across the axilla and supplies sensation to the upper medial arm and lateral upper breast (see Fig. 1-9*A*). This nerve is sometimes divided during axillary dissection, resulting in anesthesia, paresthesia, and dysesthesia of the upper medial arm. Painful neuromas may also develop as a result of intraoperative nerve injury. Care must be taken during dissection to identify and preserve the brachiocutaneous nerve as it courses between the interdigitations of the serratus an-

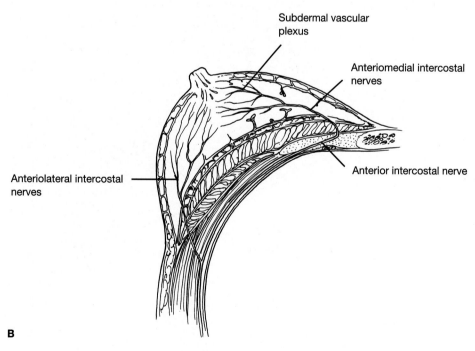

**FIGURE 1-9.**  *(Continued)*

terior muscle. Two or more separate branches of this nerve are frequently encountered.

Supraclavicular branches from the cervical plexus course beneath the platysma to innervate the upper medial breast and the overlying skin. The anterior (medial) intercostal nerves provide sensation to the medial breast and sternal areas and accompany the internal mammary perforators.

Loss of nipple sensation after breast surgery can sometimes be avoided if the surgeon understands the intraparenchymal course of the nerve supply to the nipple, the major contributor of which is the lateral branch of the fourth intercostal nerve (see Fig. 1-9*A* and *B*). This lateral branch perforates the fourth interspace at about the anterior axillary line. It travels medially under the deep fascia for 2 to 3 cm and then passes upward through the breast to supply the nipple and areola. Thus, breast resections in the mid-outer and subareolar breast are likely to alter sensation of the nipple–areolar complex. Additional contributions to innervation of the nipple may come from the third and fifth lateral intercostal nerves. The medial nipple is commonly supplied by fibers from the third through the fifth medial intercostal branches.

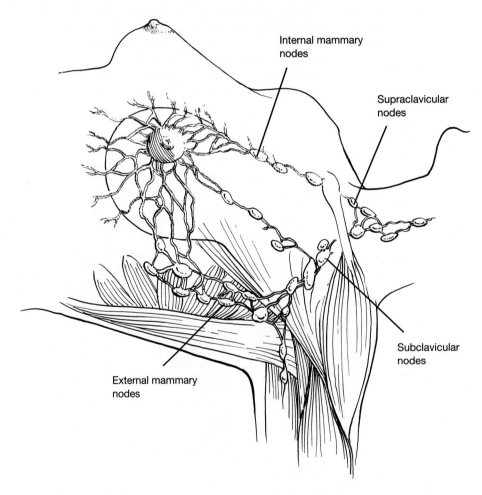

**FIGURE 1-10.** The lymphatic drainage of the breast parallels the venous flow.

### Lymphatics

Lymphatic drainage parallels the venous flow (see Fig. 1-10).[8] There are interconnecting superficial and deep lymphatic plexuses. The medial breast is drained primarily by the internal thoracic perforators to the parasternal nodes. Some lymph flows from all areas of the breast to these nodes. In the outer breast, drainage courses through the breast parenchyma around the pectoralis major and minor muscles to the subpectoral nodes. Some drainage flows directly to the subscapular chain or to the central and apical nodes of the axilla.

## ✦ SPECIAL ANATOMIC CONCERNS IN BREAST SURGERY

### Pectoral Nerves

Denervation of the pectoralis major and minor muscles contributes to significant postmastectomy deformity.[9] The resultant atrophy and loss of muscular mass complicates subsequent reconstruction. Careful dissection in the subpectoral area

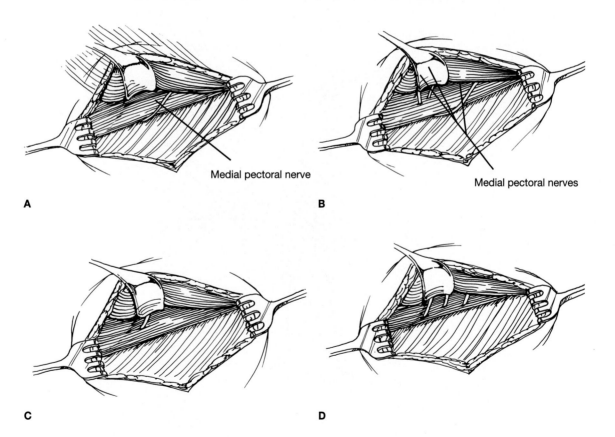

**FIGURE 1-11.** (A–D) Two to four branches of the medial pectoral nerve may course around or through the pectoralis minor muscle and overlying fat to the pectoralis major.

with identification and preservation of the medial and lateral pectoral nerves is crucial (Fig. 1-11). Two to five branches of the lateral nerve may course around or through the pectoralis minor muscle and overlying fat to the pectoralis major (see Fig. 1-11).[10]

### Thoracodorsal Neurovascular Bundle

The thoracodorsal artery, with the accompanying nerve and venae comitantes, should be preserved during the axillary dissection (Fig. 1-12). Preservation of this bundle allows subsequent use of nonatrophic latissimus dorsi muscle for breast reconstruction, should this be desirable or necessary.

If transection of the neurovascular bundle and denervation of the muscle have occurred, there may be reversal of blood flow through a serratus branch, which allows use of a viable but denervated atrophic latissimus dorsi flap (Fig. 1-13).

### Long Thoracic Nerve

The long thoracic nerve should be identified and preserved as it courses along the chest wall just posterior to the insertion of the serratus (see Fig. 1-12). Transection

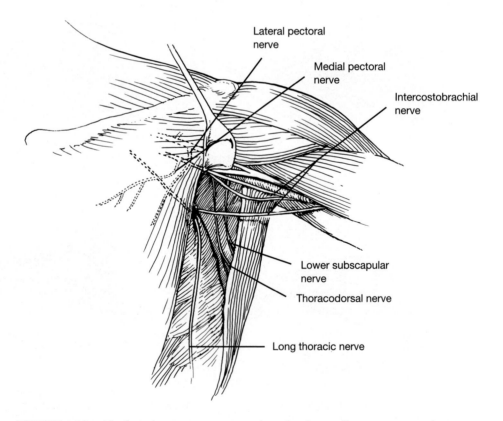

**FIGURE 1-12.** The long thoracic nerve courses along the chest wall just posterior to the insertion of the serratus anterior.

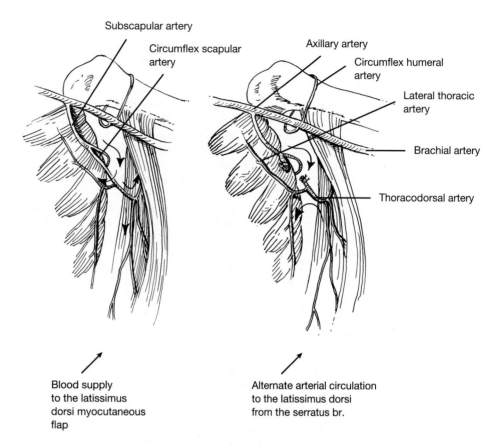

Subscapular artery

Circumflex scapular artery

Axillary artery

Circumflex humeral artery

Lateral thoracic artery

Brachial artery

Thoracodorsal artery

Blood supply
to the latissimus
dorsi myocutaneous
flap

Alternate arterial circulation
to the latissimus dorsi
from the serratus br.

**FIGURE 1-13.** If the thoracodorsal neurovascular bundle is transected, reversal of blood flow through a serratus branch may allow subsequent use of a viable but denervated latissimus dorsi.

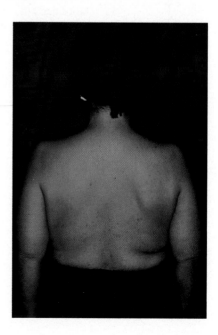

**FIGURE 1-14.** A winged right scapula caused by injury of the long thoracic nerve.

of the nerve results in winging of the scapula (Fig. 1-14), subjective weakness of the shoulder, and the related aesthetic deformity.

### *REFERENCES*

1. Braunstein GD. Gynecomastia. N Engl J Med 1993;328:490.
2. Haagensen CD. Diseases of the breast. Philadelphia: WB Saunders, 1971:2.
3. Hicken NF. Mastectomy. Clinical pathologic study demonstrating why most mastectomies result in incomplete removal of the mammary gland. Arch Surg 1940;40:6.
4. Donnegan WL, Spratt JS. Cancer of the breast. Philadelphia: WB Saunders, 1988.
5. Cooper AP. On the anatomy of the breast. London: Longmans Orme, Green, Brown, & Longmans, 1840.
5a. Sartorius OW, Morris PL, Benedict DL, Smith HS. Contrast ductography for recognition and localization of benign and malignant breast lesions: An improved technique. In: Logan WW, ed. Breast carcinoma: the radiologist's expanded role. New York: John Wiley and Sons, 1977.
5b. Noguchi S, Aihara T, Koyama H, et al. Discrimination between multicentric and multifocal carcinomas of the breast through clonal analysis. Cancer 1994;74:872.
5c. Ohuchi N, Furuta A, Mori S. Management of ductal carcinoma in situ with nipple discharge. Cancer 1994;74:1294.
6. Tinnemans JG, Lobbes T, VanderSluis RF, et al. Multicentricity in non-palpable breast carcinomas and implications for treatment. Am J Surg 1986;15:334.
7. Holland R, Veling SHJ, Mravande M, et al. Histologic multifocality of the Tis, T1-T2 breast carcinoma. Cancer 1985;56:979.
8. Holland R, Hendricks HHCL, Verbeek ALM, et al. Extent, distribution and mammographic/histological correlations of breast ductal carcinoma in situ. Lancet 1990;335:519.
9. Kinmouth JB. The lymphatics. Surgery, lymphography and diseases of the chyle and lymph system. London: Edward Arnold, 1982.
10. Serra GE, Maccarone GB, Ibarra PE, et al. Lateral pectoralis nerve: the need to preserve it in the modified radical mastectomy. J Surg Oncol 1984;26:278.
11. Moosman DA. Anatomy of the pectoral nerves and their preservation in modified mastectomy. Am J Surg 1980;139:883.

*Atlas of Techniques in Breast Surgery,*
by William Silen, W. Earle Matory, Jr. and Susan M. Love.
Lippincott-Raven Publishers, Philadelphia, © 1996.

*Chapter*

# 2

# Preservation of Breast Aesthetics: Basic Concepts

**D**eformity of the breast after diagnostic and ablative surgery results from many factors, including skin incisions or resections, parenchymal fibrosis, nipple displacement, loss of breast volume, and a change in conical shape of the breast.[1-3]

## ✦ *VARIABLE TOPOGRAPHY OF THE BREAST*

The variable topography of the human breast makes identification of resting skin tension lines (RSTL) particularly difficult. The direction and orientation of these lines may vary considerably from individual to individual, depending on the size of breast, the degree of ptosis, and the quadrant of the breast in question. Breast shape is influenced to a different degree by skin and parenchymal resection in the nine different areas of the breast (Fig. 2-1).

## ✦ *RESTING LINES OF TENSION VERSUS LANGER'S LINES*

Langer's lines[4] were derived by punching holes in the skin and assessing the direction of maximal spreading of these resultant wounds (Fig. 2-2A). Contrary to popular opinion, incisions made along Langer's lines result in spreading of the surgical scar because of the distracting forces of the underlying pectoral muscle. Resting skin tension lines are perpendicular to the direction of muscle pull. Incisions parallel to RSTLs are therefore less likely to spread. Note that Langer's lines do not coincide with lines of resting skin tension (see Fig. 2-2A through C).[5,6] In

*(text continues on p. 28)*

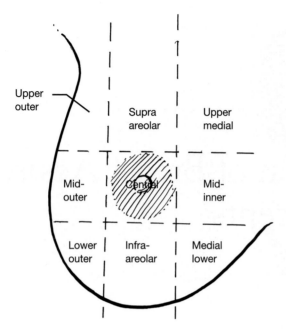

**FIGURE 2-1.** Topographic nomenclature of the breast.

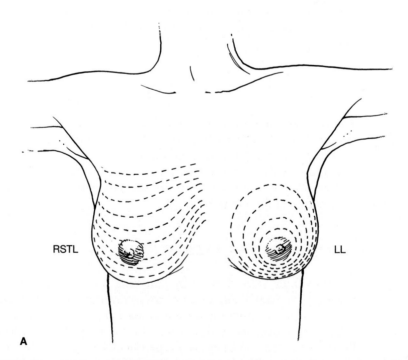

**FIGURE 2-2.** (**A**) Langer's lines (*LL*) represent lines of maximum skin tension and do not coincide with lines of resting skin tension. (**B**) Lateral and medial view of Langer's lines. (**C**) Lateral and medial view of resting skin tension lines (*RSTL*).

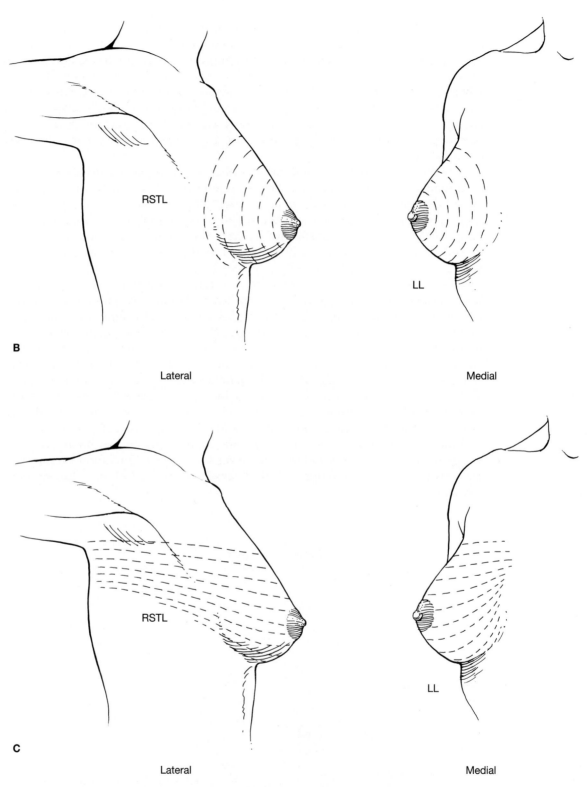

**B**

Lateral

Medial

**C**

Lateral

Medial

**FIGURE 2-2.** *(Continued)*

the upper breast, RSTLs are nearly transverse. Within the central breast, RSTLs are largely transverse, with gravity causing these lines to have a central and inferiorly directed convexity. In the lower breast, the convexity gradually becomes more parallel to the inframammary fold. Toward the tail and in the medial breast, RSTLs assume a more radial direction, ultimately fusing with the transverse axillary lines of resting skin tension. Thus, the commonly recommended circumferentially oriented breast incisions (Langer's incisions) are likely to widen and spread, producing more scarring and a less satisfactory cosmetic outcome than incisions along RSTL.

Ideally, skin incisions should parallel lines of resting skin tension, with one exception (Fig. 2-3). In the lower hemisphere of the breast, when the biopsy of an indeterminate lesion proves to be positive, elliptical resection of a transverse skin incision causes downward displacement of the nipple (even when a radial parenchymal resection is performed). Therefore, when cancer is strongly suspected, a radial skin and parenchymal resection is preferable in the lower breast (Fig. 2-4). Resections of skin and parenchyma may be shaped as an ellipse or as a wedge but elliptical incisions are preferable (Fig. 2-5*A* through *H*). In all quadrants of the breast, a radially oriented parenchymal wedge resection of the breast can achieve adequate tumor resection, preserve conical shape, and minimize nipple displacement (see Fig. 2-5*A* through *H*).[7,8] A nonradial parenchymal excision distorts the position of the nipple (see Fig. 2-5*A* through *H*). When large parenchymal excisions are anticipated, a pie-shaped wedge provides the most suitable situation for reconstruction of the breast cone. A radially oriented supra-areolar parenchymal resection is also usually most desirable because it is least likely to displace the nipple. The cutaneous scar, however, when placed radially in the supra-areolar area, is more visible and often depressed. Thus, transverse skin incisions in the RSTL are more aesthetic in the supra-areolar breast, as they are in all areas of the breast except the lower hemisphere. Radiation therapy after a properly executed wedge resection causes minimal additional fibrosis and retraction.

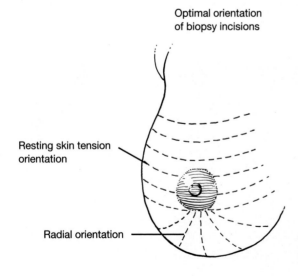

Optimal orientation
of biopsy incisions

Resting skin tension
orientation

Radial orientation

**FIGURE 2-3.** Optimal orientation of skin incisions.

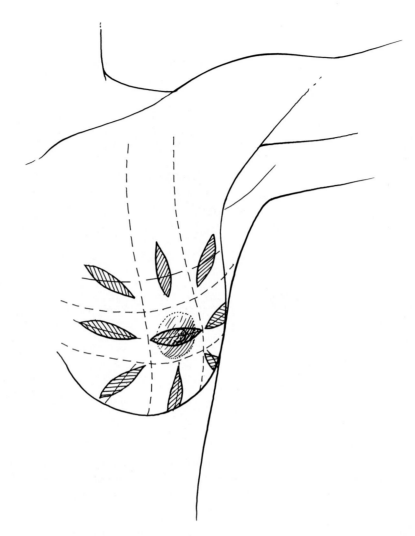

**FIGURE 2-4.**   Recommended orientation of parenchymal excision.

## ✦ *LOCATION AND EXTENT OF PARENCHYMAL RESECTION*

The location and extent of parenchymal resection influences the ultimate conical shape of the breast. The magnitude of the resection relative to the size of the breast determines the extent of change in conical configuration. In the small-breasted patient, a 2 × 2 × 2 cm resection usually results in minimal deformity. In the large breast, a 4 × 4 × 4 cm or larger resection may be equally well tolerated. Larger resections are more likely to alter the shape and volume of the breast.

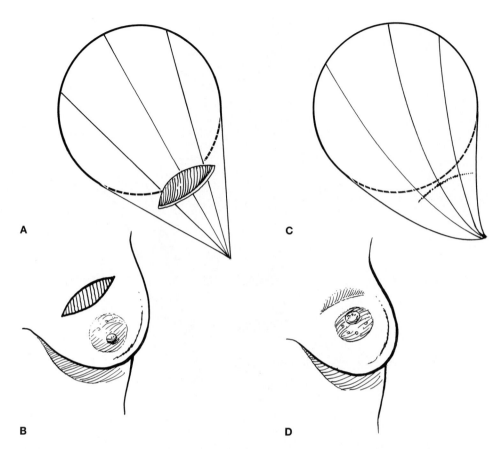

**FIGURE 2-5.** (**A–D**) A nonradial parenchymal incision distorts the ultimate position of the nipple. In this example, the areola and nipple are drawn superiorly. (**E–H**) A radial parenchymal resection does not alter the ultimate position of the nipple significantly.

## ✦ PREEXISTING POSITION OF THE BREAST OR NIPPLE

The preoperative position of the nipple (ptosis) or ptosis of the breast itself (pseudoptosis) influences the results of surgical resections. A transverse resection of skin below the nipple increases the degree of ptosis or decreases the amount of pseudoptosis (Fig. 2-6A and B). A similar resection above the nipple–areolar complex diminishes the degree of ptosis or increases pseudoptosis (see Fig. 2-6C and D). A radial resection of parenchyma does not affect the position of the nipple.[2] The optimal orientation of skin incisions for biopsy is shown in Figure 2-4.

## ✦ POSTOPERATIVE RETRACTION AND SCARRING

Increased skin tension, reactive suture material, and racial or genetic factors also influence the ultimate cosmetic outcome. In darkly pigmented patients, it is preferable to minimize the amount of absorbable suture placed in a wound because chromic

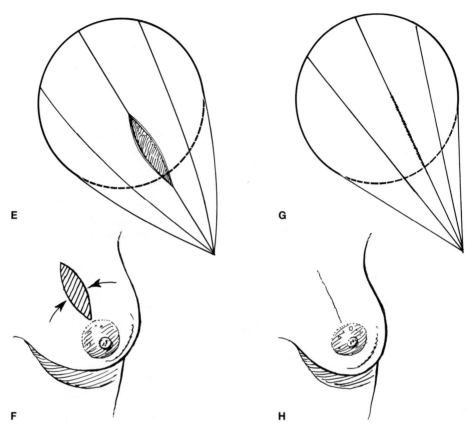

**FIGURE 2-5.** *(Continued)*

catgut and polyglycolic acid (Dexon) are highly immunoreactive. Of the commonly used absorbable sutures, polydioxanone (Vicryl) seems to be least reactive. Tamoxifen also may mitigate the cosmetic result because it increases $TGF_\beta$, which enhances fibrosis.

Fibrosis may be accentuated after seroma formation and by ischemia resulting from the surgical dissection. Radiation therapy further enhances fibrotic reaction.[2]

## ✦ ORIENTATION OF SKIN AND PARENCHYMAL RESECTIONS

Resection of skin may result in nipple displacement, depending on the location and extent of the incision and the amount of skin removed. Transverse supra- and infra-areolar parenchymal resections are most likely to displace the nipple (see Figs. 2-5 through 2-7). Medial or lateral transverse resections cause minimal displacement of the areolar complex (see Fig. 2-4). Significant nipple displacement is more likely to occur after parenchymal resections of more than 2 cm.

Surgical incisions in young or in darkly pigmented individuals have an increased propensity for hypertrophy or keloid formation. Abnormal scarring is also more

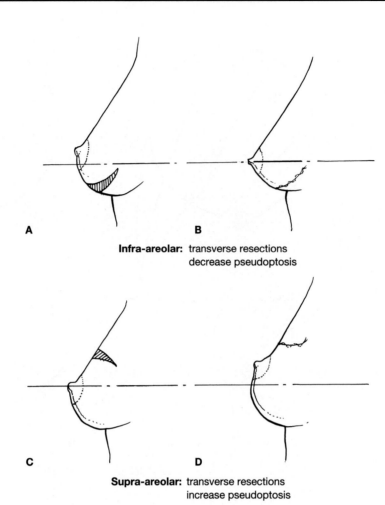

**Infra-areolar:** transverse resections
decrease pseudoptosis

**Supra-areolar:** transverse resections
increase pseudoptosis

**FIGURE 2-6.** The preoperative location of the nipple may also influence the results of surgical resections. (**A** and **B**) A transverse resection of skin below the nipple increases the degree of ptosis or decreases the degree of pseudoptosis; (**C** and **D**) A similar resection above the nipple areolar complex diminishes the degree of ptosis and increases the degree of pseudoptosis.

likely when incisions are made over the sternum; thus, mastectomy incisions should preferably not extend across the midline. Large, weighty breasts exert gravitational forces that widen surgical incisions, especially in the upper breast. In such patients, the likelihood of thickened or widened scars should be reviewed with the patient preoperatively. In contrast, circumareolar incisions rarely yield hypertrophic scarring.

The decision whether to approximate the parenchyma is influenced by several factors, including the amount of tissue resected and the location of the resection. Excisions of small amounts of breast tissue (about $1 \times 1 \times 1$ cm) rarely require closure. In the supra- and infra-areolar areas, attempted closure of a transverse excision of breast tissue produces severe distortion, whereas such is not the case medially and laterally. In most areas of the breast, a radial resection results in a gravity-induced reapproximation of the tissue. In the supra-areolar area and to a lesser extent, in the infra-areolar area, gravity causes a diastasis of the defect, and reapproximation of parenchyma is advantageous in

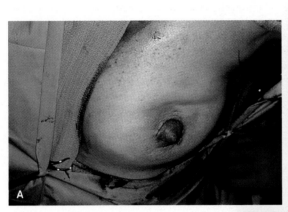
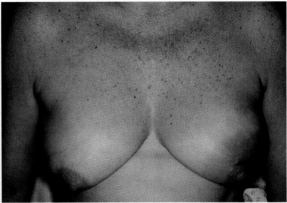
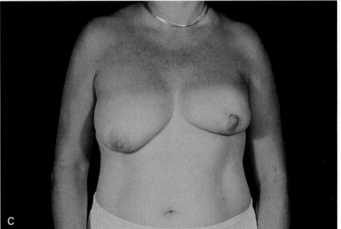

**FIGURE 2-7.** (A) A 2 × 3 × 4 cm sub- and supra-areolar resection has been performed, leaving a large defect immediately after completion of the operation. (B) Two weeks postoperatively, the defect has been obscured by a seroma creating a false sense of symmetry. (C) At completion of radiation therapy, the defect is obvious and has caused upward displacement of the nipple.

these two areas. When closure is elected, we prefer a 3-0 absorbable suture placed in fibrous parenchymal tissue, incorporating minimal fat. Tissues are approximated without strangulation. Before the completion of the operation, the head and trunk should be elevated. One can thus better assess the aesthetic outcome of parenchymal repair. One or more sutures can be released if deemed appropriate. Sometimes, the entire closure requires refashioning after removal of all of the sutures. After surgery, a bra support helps to counter the ongoing gravitational forces.

In the central breast, circumareolar, transareolar, or RSTL incisions are helpful in resecting tumor or in minimizing scarring. The lesion to be excised should be within 1 to 2 cm of the circumareolar incision. More extensive undermining compromises identification of the tumor site and increases the area of subareolar fibrosis, thus contributing to nipple displacement, distortion, and retraction.[2,3] These factors are significantly accentuated when subsequent radiation therapy is performed. Therefore, the circumareolar incision should not be used when the lesion is more than 2 cm from the areolar margin.

## REFERENCES

1. Matory WE Jr, Wertheimer M, Fitzgerald TJ, et al. Aesthetic results rollowing partial mastectomy and radiation. Plast Reconstr Surg 1990;85:739.

2. Matory WE Jr, Wertheimer M, Love S. Optimizing aesthetics following partial mastectomy. Breast Dis 1992;5:225.

3. Matory WE Jr. Partial mastectomy and radiation therapy. In: Noone B, ed. Aesthetic and reconstructive surgery of the breast. Philadelphia: BC Decker, 1991:306.

4. Langer C. Zur Anatomie and Physiologic der Haut, Sitzungsb Acad Wissench 1861;45:223.

5. Gisvold JJ, Goellner JR, Grant CS, et al. Breast biopsy: a comparative study of stereotaxically guided core and excisional techniques. Am J Roentgenol 1991;162:815.

6. Schmidt R, Morrow M, Bibbo M, et al. Benefits of stereotactic aspiration cytology. Admin Radiol 1990;9:35.

7. Layfield LJ, Chrischilles EA, Cohen MB, et al. The palpable breast nodule. A cost effectiveness analysis of alternate diagnostic approaches. Cancer 1993;72(5):1642.

8. Fornage BD. Guided fine-needle aspiration biopsy of nonpalpable breast lesions: calculation of accuracy values. Radiology 1990;177:884.

# *Part* II
# Diagnostic Procedures

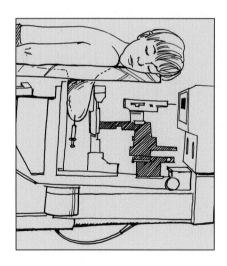

*Atlas of Techniques in Breast Surgery,*
by William Silen, W. Earle Matory, Jr. and Susan M. Love.
Lippincott-Raven Publishers, Philadelphia, © 1996.

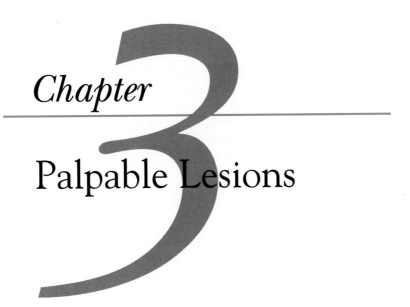

# Chapter 3

# Palpable Lesions

T he first decision any surgeon must make in evaluating the breast is whether there is an area that warrants a biopsy—that is, a dominant lump. Should one be present, the next step is to plan the best means of obtaining tissue adequate for diagnosis. Several options are available.

## ✦ FINE-NEEDLE ASPIRATION BIOPSY

This biopsy technique has been used extensively in other parts of the body but has only lately been applied to the breast. The advantage of the procedure is that it can be performed easily in the outpatient setting and yields results quickly, often within a few hours. Fine-needle aspiration biopsy does not deform the breast and does not limit future surgical options. It frequently establishes the diagnosis of malignancy and is cheaper and simpler than open biopsy.[1] For fine-needle aspiration biopsy to provide diagnostic information, an experienced cytologist must be available. The major problem with fine-needle aspiration biopsy is the potential for false-negative test results.

### Technique of Fine-Needle Aspiration Biopsy

In many centers, the cytologist rather than the surgeon performs the fine-needle aspiration biopsy. It is mandatory, however, for the surgeon to be well-acquainted with the technique and its pitfalls. Fine-needle aspiration biopsy is usually performed with a 10- or 12-mL syringe and a 21- or 23-gauge needle. Local anesthetic should be infiltrated as a wheal in the skin if desired. The operator stabilizes the lesion between his or her fingers. The needle is passed into the lesion while maintaining a vacuum on the syringe (Fig. 3-1).

Two or three passes through the lesion are made in different directions and the vacuum released before withdrawing the needle from the breast. The syringe is removed from the needle and filled with air to flush the tissue from the needle and hub.

Another method passes the needle alone into the breast, without a syringe or suction, and several passes through the lesion are conducted. The needle is withdrawn from the breast and its contents flushed into fixative or onto a side by an air-filled syringe.

The material is placed either on a slide and stained with Papanicolaou stain or fixed in 90% alcohol to be centrifuged and stained later, depending on the

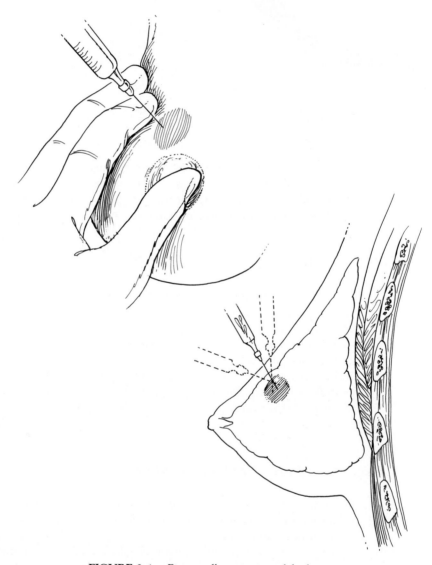

**FIGURE 3-1.** Fine-needle aspiration of the breast.

preference of the cytologist. Some surgeons prefer to use a holder or "gun" for the syringe but neither is absolutely necessary. Newer immunochemical techniques have made it possible to analyze cytologic material for estrogen receptors in addition to flow cytometry. The latter requires a special fixative and must be planned in advance.

Although the results of most series of fine-needle aspiration biopsy show it to be accurate in diagnosing breast cancer,[2,3] the overly liberal employment of fine-needle aspiration biopsy must be viewed with caution. If the number of false-positive results is high, many superfluous open operations will be recommended. It has yet to be determined whether fine-needle aspiration biopsy of every single nondominant irregularity in the breast is more cost-effective than reexamining the patient at another visit. Using fine-needle aspiration biopsy to distinguish pseudolumps from those that are truly dominant requires a close working relationship between the surgeon and the cytologist.

## *Complications*

The key disadvantage of fine-needle aspiration biopsy is the potential for false-negative test results. A negative or indeterminate cytology does not exclude the presence of cancer, and an open biopsy should be performed when there is even a remote possibility of malignancy. Most large series of fine-needle aspiration biopsy indicate that this technique has a sensitivity of about 71%, with a specificity of close to 100%.[1]

Complications of fine-needle aspiration biopsy include ecchymosis and failure to sample the lesion. Pneumothorax has been reported and is more likely to occur when the fine-needle aspiration biopsy is performed in an anesthetized patient, especially when positive-pressure ventilation is employed.

## *Rule of Concordance*

The rule of concordance is key to proper decision making. The clinical impression, mammographic interpretation, and histologic evaluation must conform with each other. Should there be any question regarding the precise diagnosis, an open biopsy must be performed. Another indication for an open biopsy is the finding of atypia in a specimen obtained by needle biopsy, in which case it is important to remove additional tissue to make certain that ductal carcinoma in situ or invasive cancer are not adjacent to the atypical area that has been sampled.

## ✦ CORE NEEDLE BIOPSIES

Core needle biopsies have been favored by some authorities over fine-needle aspiration biopsy in the United States because of the possibility of obtaining a larger sample of tissue.[4-6] In addition, core biopsy affords the option of obtaining a larger sample of tissue to analyze estrogen receptors. The disadvantages are that it is technically more difficult to perform, more painful for the patient, and may potentially sample the lesion less widely and less representatively.

### *Operative Technique*

The lesion is stabilized by the operator's nondominant hand and local anesthesia is infiltrated into the skin (Fig. 3-2). A small nick is made in the skin with a scalpel to allow the relatively large Trucut needle to enter easily. The needle is inserted into the lesion and the sheath is slid over the needle, slicing out a core of tissue.

Several cores are taken with different passes of the needle. The pressure of passing the needle is often uncomfortable but is usually tolerable. Tissue can be fixed in formalin or given fresh to the pathologist when hormone receptors are to be assessed. When the core is placed in formalin and floats rather than sinking, one has probably obtained only some fat. It is best to be certain that at least one or two cores sink.

### *Complications*

Complications include ecchymosis, hematoma, or both. The risk of pneumothorax is greater than with fine-needle aspiration because the needle is larger and the required pressure greater. Surprisingly, the false-negative rate is not much lower than with fine-needle aspiration because the tumor sometimes bounces away from the Trucut needle, particularly when it is small and mobile. Core-needle biopsies are particularly helpful in large or fixed lesions.

The golden rule for this technique and for all biopsies is that the clinical impression must match the mammographic interpretation and the histologic evaluation. Discordance of these findings should prompt an open biopsy.

### ✦ *EXCISIONAL BIOPSY*

Excisional biopsy is performed when fine-needle aspiration biopsy or core biopsy is nondiagnostic or when a small lesion requires removal. This type of biopsy, which is sometimes called lumpectomy, is used for either benign or malignant lesions. If the tumor is known or suspected to be benign (i.e., a fibroadenoma), the tumor can be removed with a minimal rim of normal tissue. Conversely, if the mass is thought or known to be malignant, it should be removed with a gross margin of about 1 cm of surrounding parenchyma. When there is doubt about the nature of a relatively large lesion, we prefer to remove a small sampling rather than an excessive amount of tissue. Reexcision can always be undertaken if necessary but it is impossible to replace normal tissue that has been removed.

The location and size of the incision is also tantamount. If the lesion is adjacent to or deep relative to the nipple, it can be removed through a circumareolar or transareolar incision. For lesions more than 1 to 2 cm from the nipple, however, we do not recommend tunneling through a circumareolar incision. The lesion may be missed and hematoma commonly occurs, as does nipple areolar distortion or displacement.

For any lesions except those bordering the nipple, we recommend a small incision along resting skin tension lines, placed directly over the palpable mass (see Fig. 2-3). For lesions farther than 1 or 2 cm from the nipple, these incisions are equally aesthetic to circumareolar ones, require less dissection, and have the additional ad-

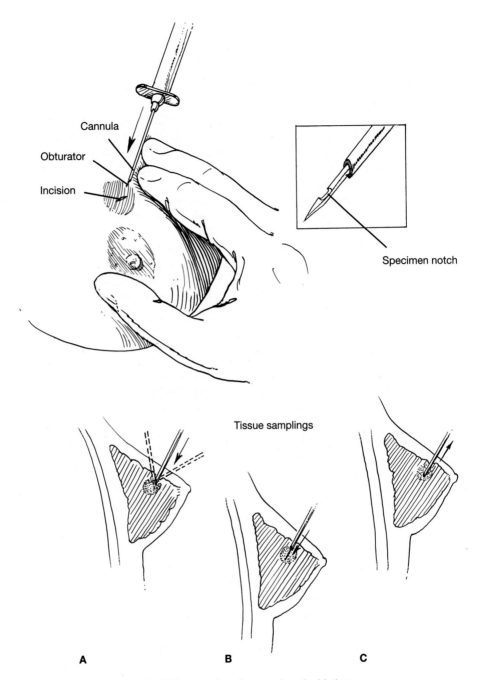

Cannula

Obturator

Incision

Specimen notch

Tissue samplings

A          B          C

**FIGURE 3-2.**   Core biopsy of a palpable lesion.

vantage of marking the location of the primary lesion should a subsequent reexcision be required.

## Operative Technique

Excisional biopsy is usually performed under local anesthesia, with or without sedation. Rarely is general anesthesia necessary. Although excisional biopsies can be performed in the office rather than in a hospital minor operating room, one must have access to a pathologist should a frozen section, hormone receptors, or ploidy analysis be desired.

The technique described below is most suitable for small lesions (up to 3 cm in diameter). Larger lesions are better managed with the techniques described for partial mastectomy (see Chap. 5).

The tumor and incision are outlined with a skin marker. Local anesthesia is infiltrated in the area of the incision and as a field block around and deep to the lesion after suitable sterile preparation and draping (Fig. 3-3*A* through *D*). The smaller the needle (30-gauge) and the slower the infiltration, the less discomfort for the patient.

### LOCAL ANESTHESIA

Lidocaine (0.5% or 1%) with $NaHCO_3$ and bupivacaine (0.25% or 0.5%) are used. Epinephrine is avoided because it provides a false sense of security regarding hemostasis. The amount of local anesthetic should be carefully monitored to stay well below toxic levels. Before beginning the incision, it is wise to test the adequacy of anesthesia by pinching the skin with forceps.

The incision is carried down through the subcutaneous fat (see Fig. 3-3*A* through *D*). Some surgeons avoid the electrocautery when removing breast lesions because the microscopic burn interferes with the evaluation of tumor margins and alters the estrogen-receptor values. When cautery is used, power should be minimized. The lesion is removed with a small rim of normal tissue and given fresh and intact to the pathologist. The specimen should be oriented for the pathologist by placing a suture at each of two locations: "long lateral, short superior" is a mnemonic that we have found to be useful.

It is our policy to give all fresh breast specimens to the pathologist immediately after excision. Bisection of the specimen by the surgeon should be avoided. Every attempt should be made to remove the specimen in one piece to allow careful pathologic review of the margins. The pathologist should stain the perimeter of the specimen with india ink before sectioning (Fig. 3-4). This technique allows margins to be identified when the permanent slides are examined. Frozen sections should not be performed; now that very small tumors are being identified, frozen sections interfere with subsequent evaluation of margins and receptor studies. Once the specimen has been removed, hemostasis is confirmed.

### PARENCHYMAL CLOSURE

Breast parenchymal approximation is seldom indicated for a *small* excisional biopsy but may be useful on other occasions. For example, in the supra-areolar breast, grav-

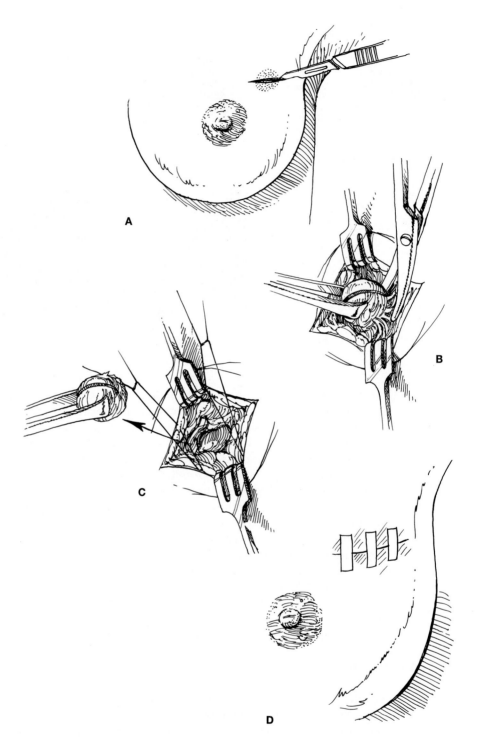

**FIGURE 3-3.** (**A–D**) Excisional biopsy. Note that skin incision in resting skin tension lines and parenchymal excision is radial.

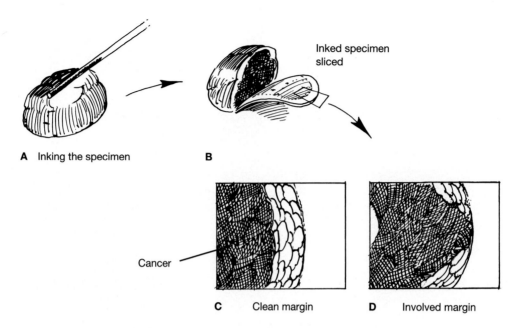

**A** Inking the specimen

**B**  Inked specimen sliced

Cancer

**C**     Clean margin        **D**     Involved margin

**FIGURE 3-4.** Handling of excisional biopsy specimen by the pathologist.

ity causes separation of the edges of a radially oriented resection, thus suggesting the need for parenchymal repair. Reapproximation of parenchyma should grasp fibrous strands (Cooper's ligaments) to close the dead space with minimal tension. The amount of incorporated fat should be minimized. After repair, the skin should be temporarily approximated. The resultant contour and tension should then be assessed in the sitting position. When distortion is noted, some or all parenchymal sutures are removed. The deep dermis is approximated with absorbable suture, and this is followed by a continuous subcuticular (intradermal) stitch. Drains are not used because they neither improve hemostasis nor prevent seromas.

When a small resection is performed anywhere in the breast or when a transverse supra-areolar resection is completed, greater distortion or nipple displacement may occur after parenchymal repair than without repair. Parenchymal reconstruction may not be indicated in the medial and lateral breast because a radial excision for parenchyma allows gravity to approximate the postresection defect, especially when a small excision has been performed.

## Complications

Complications include hematoma, infection, and seroma. Good hemostasis should avoid the former. Most excisional biopsies are relatively painless; therefore, pain in the early postoperative period requiring more than the mildest analgesic usually means that a hematoma is forming. If an acute hematoma develops, it should be evacuated in the operating room. Prophylactic antibiotics are useful to minimize the likelihood of infection when drainage of a hematoma has occurred. Postoperative seromas should be left undisturbed unless they are painful, infected, or threaten to drain spontaneously, in which case they may be aspirated with an 18- to 22-gauge needle.

## ✦ EXCISIONAL BIOPSY IN PATIENTS WITH BREAST IMPLANTS

Biopsy under this circumstance can be challenging because one must avoid injury to the prosthesis. Several precautions are advised. The patient must be introduced to the possibility of implant injury before the biopsy procedure. A plastic surgeon should be made aware of the potential need for implant replacement, thus allowing determination of the implant size and type should replacement become necessary. Electrocautery is ideal for dissection because it does not disrupt the outer envelope of the implant. In contrast, any contact with a sharp object such as scissors, a scalpel, or a needle may cause an immediate or delayed leakage. Preoperative consent must verify the willingness of the patient to accept this risk and all other potential adverse effects of biopsy (e.g., implant malposition, capsular contracture, altered breast shape or size, asymmetry, the sequelae of saline or silicone leakage, and costs of a new prosthetic device).

## ✦ EXCISIONAL BIOPSY IN THE LACTATING BREAST

Postpartum breast masses are common but definitive diagnosis is warranted. Lactation should not be a deterrent to surgery nor is surgery an indication to stop breast-feeding.

One should empty the involved breast as frequently as possible before the biopsy by bringing the infant or a breast pump to the operating suite. Excisional biopsy is undertaken, using small quantities of local anesthetic (preferably without epinephrine), and is performed in the same manner as described above for the nonlactating breast.

The lactating mother is cautioned to pump the breast for 24 hours after the procedure to prevent the ingestion of lidocaine by the infant. She should be made aware that her milk may be blood-tinged for the next few days but that breast-feeding may continue.

Galactocele or milk collections within the breast may occur postoperatively. When this occurs and is neither painful nor tense and therefore not likely to drain spontaneously, reabsorption usually occurs spontaneously. When the collection is large, tense, or painful and especially when rupture appear imminent, aspiration is indicated. Occasionally, milk fistulas develop but these invariably resolve when lactation ceases.

## ✦ INCISIONAL BIOPSY

With the increasing popularity of fine-needle aspiration and core-needle biopsies, incisional biopsies are used less frequently than in the past. Incisional biopsies are usually performed when less invasive needle biopsies are insufficient or nondiagnostic.

This procedure is also used when lesions are large or when hormone receptor levels are desired.

## *Operative Technique*

Incisional biopsies are virtually always performed under local anesthesia. The incision should be made directly over the mass and should be only as large as is necessary to obtain a representative sample of tissue (Fig. 3-5A and B).

Incisions should be placed so that the scar can be encompassed easily and without producing distortion if a partial mastectomy or modified radical mastectomy become necessary (see Chap. 5).

Once the incision is made, the subcutaneous tissue is divided to identify the tumor. When the mass is large and firm, it can be difficult to grasp with an instrument. One or two figure-of-eight sutures within the tumor may be used to stabilize the lesion. It is simplest, however, to remove a wedge with a scalpel. Once the tissue has been removed, hemostasis can be obtained with electrocautery or hemostatic sutures. Parenchymal reapproximation is rarely indicated after incisional biopsy because the rigid unyielding tumor tissue makes it virtually impossible to accomplish. The deep dermis is closed with absorbable suture and the skin with a subcuticular continuous suture.

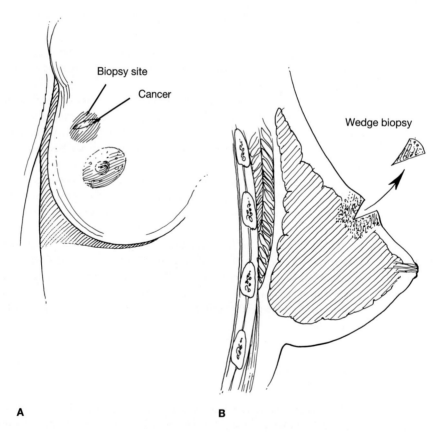

**A**

**B**

**FIGURE 3-5.** Incisional biopsy.

## *Complications*

The most common pitfall in the performance of an incisional biopsy is the harvest of insufficient tissue for diagnosis and for determination of hormone receptors or the presence of tumor markers. The margin of the tumor is sometimes fibrotic or necrotic and may not yield enough material for diagnosis unless a more central part of the lesion is sampled. Fine-needle aspiration biopsy or core-needle biopsy can be performed through an open incision when necessary to obtain deeper or more definitive specimens.

### *REFERENCES*

1. Layfield LJ, Chrischilles EA, Cohen MB, et al. The palpable breast nodule. A cost effectiveness analysis of alternate diagnostic approaches. Cancer 1993;72(5):1642.
2. Kopans DB. Fine-needle aspiration of clinically occult breast lesions. Radiology 1989;170:313.
3. Martelli G, Pilotti S, de Yoldi G, et al. Diagnostic efficacy of physical examination, mammography, fine needle aspiration cytology (triple test) in solid breast lumps: an analysis of 1708 consecutive cases. Tumori 1990;76:476.
4. Burbank F, Belville J. Core breast biopsy, research, and what not to do. Radiology 1992;185:639.
5. Parker SH. When is core biopsy really core? Radiology 1992;185:641.
6. Foster RS. Core-cutting needle biopsy for the diagnosis of breast cancer. Am J Surg 1982;143:622.

*Atlas of Techniques in Breast Surgery,*
by William Silen, W. Earle Matory, Jr. and Susan M. Love.
Lippincott-Raven Publishers, Philadelphia, © 1996.

# Chapter 4

# Nonpalpable Lesions

ass screening mammography has resulted in the detection of greatly increased numbers of very small breast lesions.

## ✦ STEREOTACTIC BIOPSY

Mammographically guided stereotactic breast biopsy is performed with the patient in the supine position and with the breast fixed in the mammography machine. The radiograph tubes are angled at about 15 degrees from the central axis. The tumor location can thus be precisely identified relative to a fixed reference grid, allowing four to five passes of either a 25-gauge needle into the mass to obtain material for cytologic examination (stereotactic fine-needle aspiration) or a 14-gauge needle that obtains a core of tissue (stereotactic core-needle biopsy). A digital mammogram is used to confirm the column of air traversing the lesion and thus, tumor localization. Localization accuracy is excellent to within 2 mm (Fig. 4-1).

### Efficacy of Stereotactic Breast Biopsy

Experience with stereotactic breast biopsy throughout the United States[1,2] suggests that experienced operators can yield interpretable specimens (sufficient samples) nearly 100% of the time.

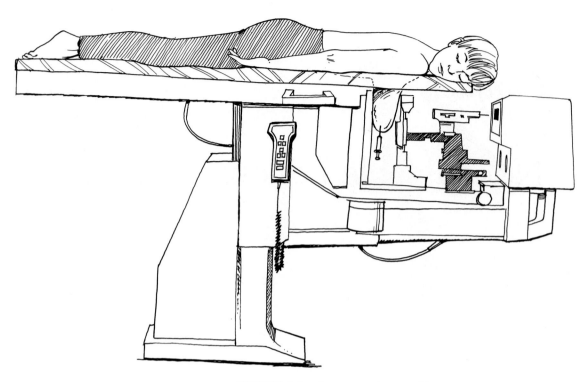

**FIGURE 4-1.** Stereotactic biopsy table.

## Indications

Stereotactically guided breast biopsy is ideal for sampling nonpalpable breast lesions. Stereotactic biopsy techniques are not especially suitable for small areas of calcification or for lesions that are superficial or located in the perimeter of the breast. Stereotactic techniques have about halved the cost of excisional biopsy.[3,4]

To improve the incidence of definitive diagnoses using stereotactic techniques, core-biopsy devices can obtain sufficient tissue for diagnosis in 99.7% of cases in experienced hands.[2] The yield of needle biopsies in providing a definitive diagnosis can eliminate 50% of open surgical biopsies.[1] The complication rate of 0.2% bespeaks the safety of this technique. General pathologists are more comfortable interpreting the histologic specimens after core biopsy, and inconclusive reports that often accompany stereotactic fine-needle aspiration are less frequent with a core. The size of the core can be accurately judged by the human eye, thus shortening the learning curve of the surgeon for stereotactic core biopsy in comparison with fine-needle aspiration biopsy (FNAB).

## Pros and Cons

The potential for misdiagnosis of borderline atypia or for missing areas of microinvasion remains a drawback to stereotactic fine-needle aspiration. Thus, patients with suspicious or atypical lesions by either FNAB or core biopsy should undergo open biopsy. When malignancy is diagnosed on the FNAB, cytology has a low false-positive rate but it is not zero.[5]

Core biopsy can identify invasion and false-negative results are infrequent.[1,5,6] Core biopsy results compare almost perfectly with the results of open biopsy.[6] Complete agreement between the results of stereotactic core biopsy with a 14-gauge needle and open biopsy can be obtained.[7] An FNAB fails to produce a definitive diagnosis in 27% to 50%, whereas the incidence of failure to produce a definitive diagnosis with core biopsy can approach zero.

One of the key advantages of stereotactic FNAB and core biopsy is the absence of any lasting postbiopsy changes on the skin and on the mammogram. Scarring after excisional biopsy is eliminated, thus enhancing the accuracy of mammographic follow-up.

The yield of needle biopsies that provide enough information to allow definitive treatment can result in the elimination of 50% of open surgical biopsies.[7] As a result, cost-savings in breast cancer diagnosis will be tremendous. Stereotactic biopsy techniques safely, effectively, and less expensively enhance diagnostic capabilities for nonpalpable lesions.[7]

## ✦ WIRE LOCALIZATION AND OPEN BIOPSY

Wire localization biopsy is employed when stereotactic core biopsy is not indicated, is not available, or is indeterminate. It is important that the surgeon and radiologist discuss the case before the procedure, both to agree on the necessity for the technique and to review the best possible approach. Because the goal is to excise the tumor without removing a large amount of additional tissue, the localization must be precise (within 0.5 cm of the lesion). Several needle and wire combinations are available. We find the hook wire (Kopans) or the Sadowski wire preferable because they have a smaller tip that allows more precise dissection. Both come with a stiffener or shaft that can be passed over the wire to make it palpable. The curved wire (Homer)[8] is technically easier to use for the inexperienced radiologist but the wire encompasses a large amount of breast tissue and thus necessitates larger biopsies. Some centers use dye as a marker, either in addition to or as an alternative to wire. Skin markers alone are not sufficiently accurate because a single needle or even two straight needles on the skin have the risk of displacement as the patient moves from the radiology department to the operating suite.

Most radiologists prefer to insert the wire from the superior or lateral position, parallel to the chest wall. Although it would be easier for the surgeon if the wire were inserted directly in and through the lesion along the same path as the proposed incision, this is technically more difficult for the radiologist and more likely to decrease the accuracy of localization.

It is crucial that localization be precise and within 5 mm of the lesion. A localization more than 1 cm from the lesion is inadequate and unacceptable. Once the wire has been placed in the breast, the patient is brought to the operating room.

## Operative Technique

Most wire localization biopsies are performed under local anesthesia, even when the lesion is "deep" or within a large breast. Short-acting general anesthetic agents provide the surgeon and anesthesiologist with an additional method to improve patient comfort.

The entry site of the wire through the skin and its relation to the tip of the wire determines the optimal surgical approach. Generally, it is wise to estimate from the radiograph and the position of the wire the position of the tip of the wire within the breast. One must keep in mind that the patient is in a far different position during the localization procedure than on the operating table (seated leaning forward in the radiology suite and lying supine in the operating room), significantly changing relation of the tumor to the wire. A radio-opaque marker placed at the border of the areola and at the entry site of the wire can be helpful in orienting the surgeon. Sometimes, gently palpating the breast while watching the direction of movement of the wire reveals the position of the tip within the breast (Fig. 4-2A). It is not wise to exert traction on the wire because this may dislodge it. Once a decision has been made regarding the position of the end of the wire, the surgeon can mark the skin and outline the desired incision.

We suggest placing the incision along resting skin tension lines as close to the lesion as possible to minimize dissection and to simplify identification of the biopsy site should a future reexcision be necessary. When the lesion is superficial or when the

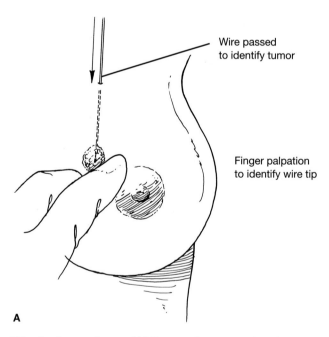

Wire passed
to identify tumor

Finger palpation
to identify wire tip

**A**

**FIGURE 4-2.** Wire localization biopsy. (**A**) Finger palpation to identify wire tip. (**B**) Local infiltration and incision. (**C**) Dissection to identify the needle hub. (**D**) End of the wire is grasped. (**E**) End of wire is pulled into the biopsy site. (**F**) Tumor with surrounding breast is removed with the wire hook embedded.

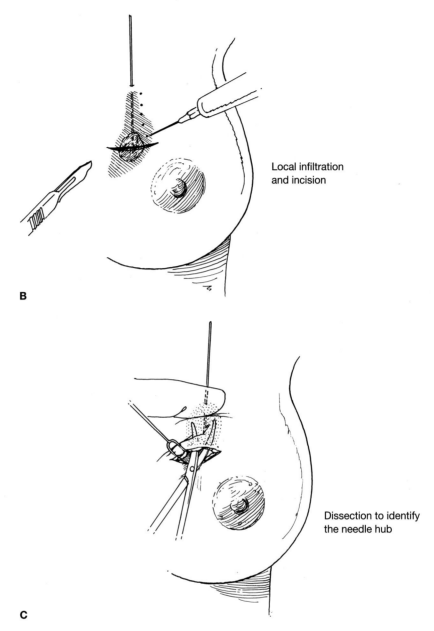

Local infiltration
and incision

**B**

Dissection to identify
the needle hub

**C**

**FIGURE 4-2.** *(Continued)*

wire points directly and posteriorly into the breast, the incision may encompass the entry site of the wire. Otherwise, the incision is better placed further along the path of the wire (see Fig. 4-2*A*). After infiltration with lidocaine, the skin is incised along resting skin tension lines. The subcutaneous fat is separated until the wire is identified (see Fig. 4-2*B* and *C*).

It is often helpful to cut the protruding cutaneous end of the wire at this point and pass it into the incision (see Fig. 4-2*D*). The tissue surrounding the wire is grasped with an Allis clamp and dissected along the wire (see Fig. 4-2*E*). Additional

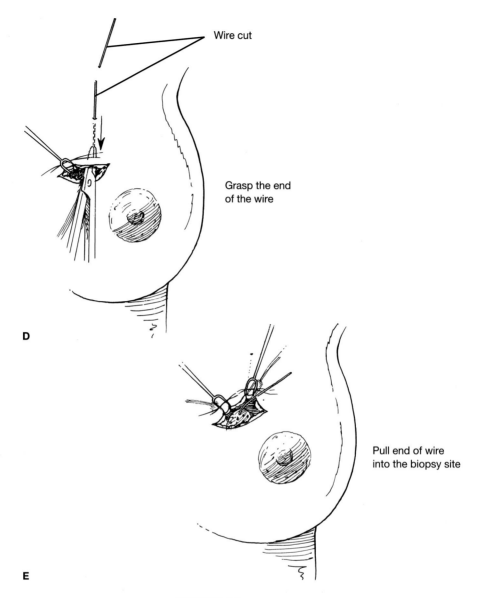

**FIGURE 4-2.**  *(Continued)*

local anesthetic may be required as the exact area to be dissected becomes apparent. Once the lesion is removed, a radiograph of the specimen is taken.

The injection of blue dye around the lesion by the radiologist before the wire is placed may reduce the incidence of failure to remove the mammographic lesion. Many surgeons prefer the use of dye to wire localization. A needle is used to localize the lesion as described above and then a vital dye containing iodinated contrast material is injected into the tissue. Excision of the stained area may be a little more difficult when dye alone without a needle is used because there is no cutaneous landmark to help the surgeon locate the area in question (e.g., the entrance of the wire into the breast).

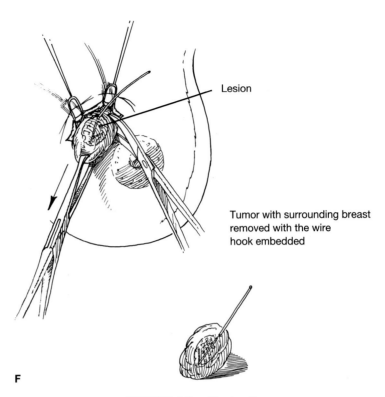

Lesion

Tumor with surrounding breast
removed with the wire
hook embedded

F

FIGURE 4-2. (*Continued*)

If the lesion is not removed in the initial excision, further attempts may result in removal of an excessive volume of the breast tissue in a relatively indiscriminate manner. Precise localization is therefore essential. Only one further attempt at excision of the lesion is suggested when the lesion or microcalcifications are not present on the specimen mammogram. In rare instances in which calcifications have been missed, it is easier to again attempt radiologic localization 6 weeks later.

## ✦ KEY CONSIDERATIONS

Large resections defeat the purpose and advantage of discovering small nonpalpable lesions. We cannot overemphasize the importance of minimizing the amount of tissue that is removed. Attempts to obtain tumor-free margins are ill-advised as part of the *initial* wire localization procedure. This operation is designed to be strictly diagnostic.

Once the specimen has been removed and radiographed, hemostasis is confirmed. Some surgeons believe that it is preferable to avoid electrocautery when removing breast tumors because it makes interpretation of the margins more difficult. Because reexcision of a malignant lesion is often indicated, the issue may be of limited significance. Breast tissue should be approximated or left unapproximated, according to the discussion in Chapter 5. The dermis is closed, and the skin is approximated with a subcuticular suture. Drains are not indicated.

Ultrasound, magnetic resonance imaging, and computed tomography scans have been used in addition to mammography to localize small tumors. These techniques are particularly helpful when the breast mass cannot be identified in two mammographic views because of the curved contour of the chest wall.

### Specimen Mammography

The specimen mammogram determines whether the lesion has been sampled, as does a follow-up mammogram of the patient within 3 to 6 weeks. The latter is particularly helpful when the findings on the specimen mammogram are equivocal and may also identify residual calcifications or other suspicious findings. Surgical clips may be placed along the retained margins of the biopsy site. This may be useful for the radiation therapist or for a future reexcision if the lesion is found to be malignant; however, because 70% to 80% of nonpalpable lesions are benign, clips are best reserved for the time of definitive resection.

### Complications

Failure to excise the occult lesion is one of the most common pitfalls of wire localization. Patients should be informed of this potential risk preoperatively. The best way to avoid this risk is to accept only precise localization. Compensating for a suboptimal localization by removing a large amount of breast tissue is a disservice to the patient and defeats the purpose of early detection and localization. In our opinion, if the lesion is not present in the specimen, the best tactic is to repeat the entire procedure in 6 to 12 weeks.

Another untoward event is that of retention of a portion of the wire, which usually occurs when the stem of the wire is cut prematurely. This was more common with the early versions of hook wires, which were thin and easy to cut. If a piece of wire is retained within the breast, it may be left or it may be localized and retrieved. If allowed to remain, the patient must be informed of the presence of the wire and concomitant risks.

Poor diagnostic planning that results in removal of a large breast volume may make cosmetic reexcision difficult or impossible. If the lesion is malignant and breast conservation is elected, a reexcision is almost invariably required to obtain tumor-free margins. A large preexisting defect may make breast conservation impossible, thus condemning the patient to mastectomy. Another concern arises when reexcision is required in a patient whose initial cutaneous incision is far removed from the tumor. The surgeon is then required to estimate as nearly as possible the location of the tumor, a difficult task at best. We recommend that the incision be made as close to the lesion as possible and that the smallest amount of tissue required to make the diagnosis be removed.

## ✦ DEFINITIVE RESECTION OF NONPALPABLE MASSES

As noninvasive techniques are used increasingly to diagnose nonpalpable lesions, the initial surgical procedure may be definitive rather than solely diagnostic. The technique used for the definitive resection of a nonpalpable lesion differs from that of the removal of tissue for diagnostic purposes. A definitive resection using multiple wires is described in Chapter 5.

### *REFERENCES*

1. Gisvold JJ, Goellner JR, Grant CS, et al. Breast biopsy: a comparative study of stereotaxically guided core and excisional techniques. Am J Roentgenol 1991;162:815.
2. Jackson VP. The status of mammographically guided fine needle aspiration biopsy of nonpalpable breast lesions. Radiol Clin North Am 1992;30:155.
3. Parker SH. Percutaneous large core breast biopsy. Cancer 1994;74(Suppl):256.
4. Schmidt R, Morrow M, Bibbo M, et al. Benefits of stereotactic aspiration cytology. Admin Radiol 1990;9:35.
5. Fornage BD. Guided fine-needle aspiration biopsy of nonpalpable breast lesions: calculation of accuracy values. Radiology 1990;177:884.
6. Dowlatshahi K, Yaremko ML, Kluskens LF, et al. Nonpalpable breast lesions: findings of stereotaxic needle-core biopsy and fine-needle aspiration cytology. Radiology 1991; 181:745.
7. Kopans DB. Review of stereotaxic large-core needle biopsy and surgical biopsy results in non-palpable breast lesions. Radiology 1993;189:665.
8. Homer MJ, Smith TJ, Safaii H. Prebiopsy needle localization: methods, problems and expected results. Radiol Clin North Am 1992;30:139.

# *Part* *III*

# Strategies in the Surgical Treatment of Malignant Disease

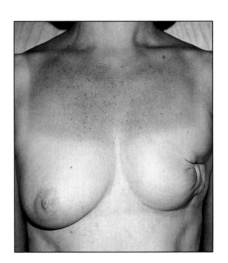

*Atlas of Techniques in Breast Surgery,*
by William Silen, W. Earle Matory, Jr. and Susan M. Love.
Lippincott-Raven Publishers, Philadelphia, © 1996.

*Chapter* 5

# Partial Mastectomy

The goals of breast conservation are (1) removal of tumor mass with a margin of normal surrounding tissue, achieving a cosmetic outcome that is acceptable to the patient, and (2) preservation of sensibility when possible. Many terms have been used to describe limited resection of the breast for the treatment of carcinoma. These include lumpectomy, wide local excision, segmental resection, quadrantectomy, segmental tylectomy, reexcision, and partial mastectomy. None of these descriptions, except possibly quadrantectomy, define the amount of tissue that is to be removed. We prefer to use the term "partial mastectomy" to define myriad procedures that potentially alter the size, shape, and contours of the breast.

The precise amount of normal breast tissue that should be resected around a malignant lesion is not known. Although quadrant excision and radiation therapy produce results equivalent to those of mastectomy in terms of survival and a low incidence of local recurrence,[1] quadrantectomy sometimes removes more tissue than necessary, which may compromise the cosmetic result.

Several factors increase the risk of local failure after partial mastectomy and radiation. Microscopic evaluation of inked margins is admittedly crude and only provides a gross estimate of whether margins are involved.[2] A pathologist can evaluate only small samples of the perimeter of the specimen under optimal conditions.[2] To examine the entire perimeter of a 2-cm tumor would require the processing of at least 2000 slides. Thus, conventional assessment of margin involvement is not precise. Histologic characteristics of the tumor may be of greater value in dictating the extent of resection.[3] When the tumor is a sclerotic infiltrating ductal carcinoma, the lesion can be removed with a small rim (1 cm) of normal tissue, with the expectation that there will be little residual disease. Conversely, when the tumor is less well-localized (e.g., an infiltrating lobular carcinoma) or when an extensive intraductal component is present, a larger volume of resection is indicated, accompanied by a careful microscopic inspection of the margins. An infiltrating ductal carcinoma with an extensive intraductal component (i.e., ductal carcinoma in situ with tumor extension) creates additional concerns. In this circumstance, the difficulty in ascertaining whether the cancer has been removed entirely is magnified. Although the presence of ductal carcinoma in situ at the margin of resection is not universally interpreted as being pathologically significant, our studies[3,4] and those of others[5,6] indicate that extensive ductal carcinoma in situ in association with an infiltrative lesion is associated with a high incidence of local recurrence after excision and radiation therapy, especially if the margins are not clear. A more generous resection, with close attention to involvement of margins, with ductal carcinoma in situ indicates whether the patient can be safely treated with radiation (clear margins) or whether the extensive ductal carcinoma in situ requires mastectomy.[7]

## ✦ AESTHETIC CONSIDERATIONS OF PARTIAL MASTECTOMY

The other crucial component of breast conservation is the ability to remove the cancer without disfiguring the remaining breast. Aesthetic outcome after partial mastectomy is primarily influenced by:

1. Size of resection relative to the size of the breast
2. Location of the tumor and the tumor resection within the breast
3. Orientation of the skin and parenchymal resections
4. Postsurgical and postradiation scar retraction

Only the latter two factors can be influenced by surgical techniques that optimize cosmesis.

### Size of Resection Relative to Breast Size

In small or medium-sized breasts (less than 1000 g/D cup), large resections result in significant aesthetic deformity (Fig. 5-1). This deformity may be further compounded by radiation-induced retraction in some patients.

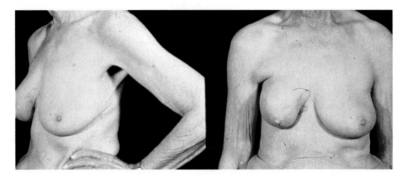

**FIGURE 5-1.** A significant deformity occurs after a sizable resection in a medium-sized breast.

Resections of more than 25% of the breast volume in small or medium-sized breasts should be avoided in most cases. Total mastectomy, with or without reconstruction, may yield a more attractive outcome in such cases. In the large-breasted patient having considerable redundancy of parenchyma and skin (more than 1000 g/DD cup or greater), large partial mastectomies of up to 50% to 60% can be accomplished aesthetically using plastic surgical breast reduction techniques. In large breasts, wedge resections with minimal undermining allow preservation of blood supply and satisfactory cosmetic outcomes after breast conservation.

## Location of Tumor and Tumor Resection

Some of the least aesthetic outcomes after partial mastectomy occur after resections in the supra-areolar, the upper inner, and the mid-medial breast. These are the thinner areas of the breast, in which parenchymal resections are more likely to demonstrate the resultant volume reduction than any other regions. Such resections result in either a soft-tissue depression (Fig. 5-2*A*) or in an elevation of nipple height (see Fig. 5-2*B*).

In contrast, partial resections in the upper outer, mid-lateral, lower lateral, central, infra-areolar, and lower medial breast consistently yield satisfactory cosmetic outcomes (Fig. 5-3*A* through *D*).

## Orientation of Skin and Parenchymal Resections

Aesthetic concerns bring forth many additional factors that must be entertained in surgical planning. Many of these have been outlined in Chapters 2 and 3.[8,9] In most areas of the breast, skin incisions should be parallel to lines of resting skin tension.

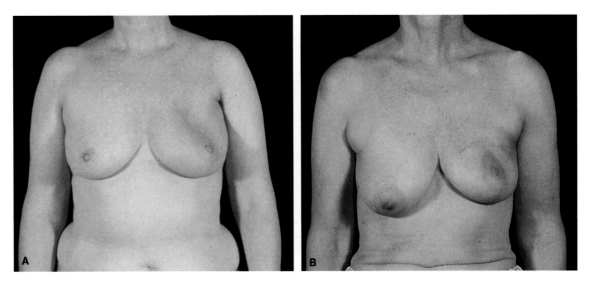

**FIGURE 5-2.**    (**A**) A resection in the upper inner area has resulted in a soft tissue depression. (**B**) A supra-areolar resection often results in elevation of the nipple.

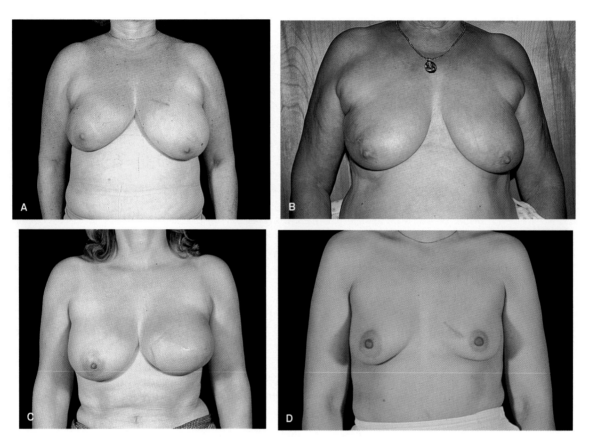

**FIGURE 5-3.** Skin and parenchymal resection from areas of the breast other than supra-areolar areas can result in an acceptable cosmetic outcome. Each patient is depicted 1 year or longer after partial mastectomy and a 6-week course of 54–65 Gy of external beam, with or without electron boost therapy. (**A**) After 6 × 7 × 10 cm resection from the upper inner breast. (**B**) A 7 × 6 × 8 cm resection from the mid-lateral outer area, resulting in minimal deformity. (**C**) After a 12 × 6 × 8 cm resection of the central left breast. (**D**) After a 2 × 4 × 5 cm removal from the medial breast.

In the lower hemisphere of the breast, the disadvantage of skin incisions along resting skin tension lines (RSTLs) is that if a reexcision of this transverse resection should be required, the nipple becomes displaced inferiorly. Therefore, in the lower half of the breast, skin and parenchymal resections should be both radial to the nipple and should be shaped as an ellipse (Fig. 5-4A and B) or as a wedge.

In all quadrants of the breast, a radially oriented parenchymal wedge resection minimally alters the conical shape and results in little nipple displacement (see Fig. 5-4A and B). When large excisions are anticipated, a pie-shaped wedge of breast parenchyma provides the most suitable design for reconstruction of the breast cone (see Fig. 5-4C and D). Radiation therapy after a properly executed wedge resection causes minimal additional fibrosis and retraction. A radially oriented supra-areolar parenchymal resection is least likely to displace the nipple but a radial cutaneous scar is more visible than a transverse incision. Consequently, the ideal procedure in the supra-areolar area is a skin incision in the RSTL (almost transverse), coupled with a radial parenchymal excision. A transverse resection of supra-areolar parenchyma

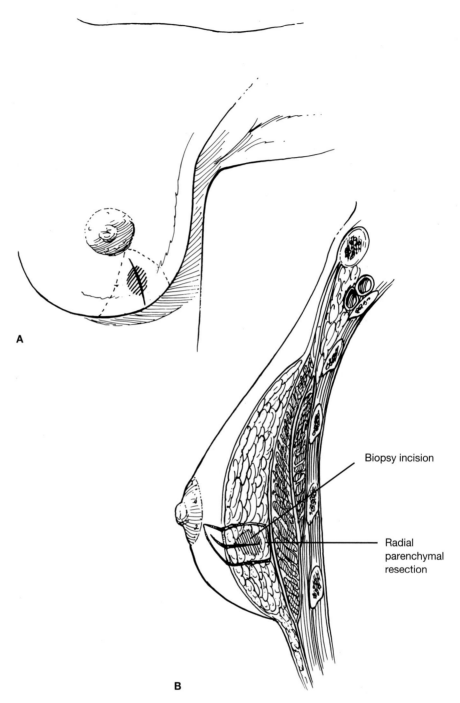

Biopsy incision

Radial
parenchymal
resection

A

B

**FIGURE 5-4.** (A–D) Partial mastectomy. Note the radial parenchymal excision.

*(continued)*

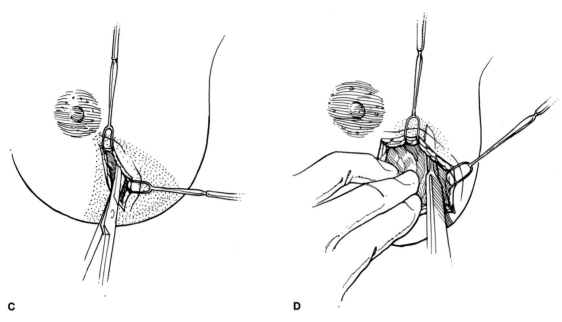

C                                    D

**FIGURE 5-4.** *(Continued)*

raises the nipple. In contrast, a supra-areolar radial resection of parenchyma causes minimal nipple displacement of the areola.

In the central breast, circumareolar or transareolar incisions, with or without extensions along RSTL, are helpful in minimizing scarring. The lesion to be excised through such incisions should be within 1 to 2 cm of the outer rim of the areola. More extensive undermining increases the area of subareolar fibrosis and contributes to nipple displacement, distortion, and retraction. Fibrosis, retraction, distortion, and displacement are significantly enhanced after radiation therapy. Therefore, the circumareolar incision should not be used when the lesion is more than 1 to 2 cm from the areolar margin.

Nipple areolar involvement with cancer is likely when lesions are within 2 cm of the areola,[10] implying the need for centric resection.

Centric resection with removal of the nipple–areolar complex maintains excellent breast contour. Nipple reconstruction can be performed subsequently.

In the lower breast, removal of a significant amount of breast tissue can be accomplished aesthetically by removing breast tissue in a pie-shaped wedge, with the apex oriented to the nipple.

## Postsurgical and Postradiation Retraction

Fibroblastic proliferation is incited by surgical trauma and by radiation injury. Seromas may contribute to the ultimate formation of excessive scarring. Radiation therapy causes obliteration of blood vessels and may accentuate postsurgical scarring, so that retraction or nipple displacement may result (see Fig. 5-5A and B). Edema and induration are most prominent within the first 12 to 24 months but scarring persists and may progress over many years.

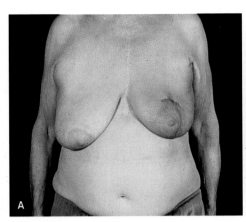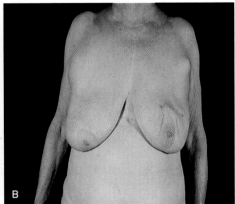

**FIGURE 5-5.** (**A**) This 65-year-old woman is shown after a 4 × 4 × 5 cm supra-areolar resection, 1 month after completion of 58 Gy by external beam. She demonstrates erythema, induration, tenderness, telangiectasia, peau d'orange, and retraction. (**B**) Fifteen months later, additional retraction and uplifting of the areola has occurred, with resolution of most of the acute symptoms.

Wide undermining augments seroma formation and fibroblastic proliferation and should be avoided. This excessive trauma prolongs the inflammatory response, in addition to compromising patient comfort and the aesthetic outcome.

Wide undermining associated with partial or total mastectomy, level II or II axillary dissection along with chest wall, or axillary radiation may contribute to severe and permanent soft-tissue and joint fibrosis.

Hemostasis must be absolute and technique must be as gentle as possible at the time of partial mastectomy. Most surgeons do not drain the cavity that is produced by a partial mastectomy because drains do not prevent seromas and may enhance the chances of infection.

## ✦ OPERATIVE TECHNIQUE

A skin marker is used to outline the tumor and surrounding normal breast to encompass the tumor with a 1-cm margin. When a reexcision is performed, ideally the previous scar should be resected. When resection of the scar is anticipated to produce a less than optimal aesthetic outcome, one may choose to use a new and separate incision. Most of these patients receive postoperative radiation and both scars can be given a radiation boost, if necessary.

Flaps of skin and subcutaneous fat of at least 1 cm in thickness are elevated medially and laterally (see Fig. 5-4*C*). Electrocautery is not used by some surgeons to avoid compromise of the pathologic assessment of the margins, although this drawback is probably overemphasized. Once the borders of the proposed excision have been reached, the resection proceeds to the level of the pectoralis muscle. Care must be taken at this point to carry the plane of dissection perpendicular to the chest wall to prevent inadvertently removing more tissue than planned.

The specimen is dissected from the pectoralis muscle, including pectoralis fascia, as the deep margin of resection. If the deep side of the specimen is adherent to the muscle, a portion of muscle is also removed, thus providing the same deep margin as would be expected in a mastectomy.

Once the specimen is removed, it is carefully oriented for the pathologist by placing two marking sutures. A drawing of the breast and the surgical specimen on a towel further clarifies and orients the breast mass for the pathologist. Frozen-section assessment of the margins is deemed inappropriate in most cases because detailed analysis of the margins by this means is not feasible. If the pathologist finds that the gross margins are involved, more tissue should be resected.

### Approximation of Breast Parenchyma

Whether one performs postresection reapproximation of the breast parenchyma depends on the location within the breast and the volume of the defect. After a large resection relative to the size of the breast (more than 20%), the deformity that results from reapproximating parenchyma may be worse than the unapproximated defect.

In most areas of the breast, a radial resection results in a gravity-induced reapproximation of tissue, so that internal suture approximation of breast tissue is unnecessary, although not adverse. In the supra-areolar breast, and to a lesser extent in the infra-areolar area, gravity causes a diastasis of the wound edges. Reapproximation of parenchyma is appropriate in these two locations (Fig. 5–6).

Generally, women assess their cosmetic result while looking in the mirror in the standing position. In our experience, most women tolerate a visible deformity in the

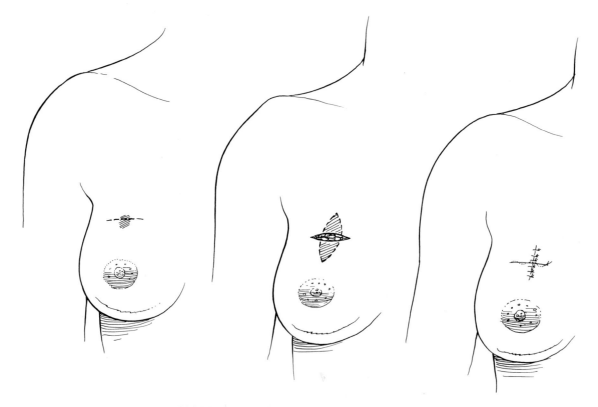

**FIGURE 5-6.** Closure of the breast parenchyma.

supine position if the breast is well-contoured when the patient is upright. The decision to reapproximate the breast and the manner of approximation should be analyzed with gravitational forces in mind. After approximating the skin edges, the patient's breast is evaluated in the sitting position, with and without parenchymal closure (Fig. 5-7). If breast contour and symmetry are acceptable without closure, approximation may be omitted. Although revision can be performed at a later date, it is desirable to avoid it by carefully evaluating the appearance at the time of operation.

If closure of breast tissue is elected, the parenchyma along one edge of the operative defect is grasped loosely with Allis clamps and dissected subcutaneously, elevating a skin flap of 1 cm or thicker. A similar procedure is performed on both sides of the defect. We prefer a 2-0 or 3-0 absorbable suture placed in fibrous parenchyma, incorporating minimal fat. Tissues should be approximated without strangulation. Two layers are used to appose the breast tissue closest to the nipple, thus reforming the breast cone. As the closure proceeds away from the nipple, the breast tapers and becomes thinner and only one layer of parenchymal closure is necessary. Temporary skin staples or sutures are used to approximate skin. The breast contour is then checked again in the sitting position. If dimpling, depressions, or contour deformity are noted, sutures can be removed or repositioned to optimize shaping. If the apex of the incision is at the areola, it may be necessary to carry the incision around the areola for a short distance to eliminate contour irregularity. Drains are usually not required. After surgery, bra support helps to counter adverse gravitational forces. A sample outcome is illustrated (Fig. 5-8).

Even the most aesthetic parenchymal approximation after partial mastectomy defect may not stand the test of time. Avulsion of the parenchymal repair may occur (possibly as a result of postsurgical or postsuture devascularization), leaving the original postresection defect. Experience has led one of the authors to leave large resections without reapproximation, whereas another goes to great lengths to close the defect.

Regardless, two principles should be given special attention:

1.   Avoid tension at the site of any repair of parenchymal tissue.
2.   Check breast size, shape, and contour in the sitting position.

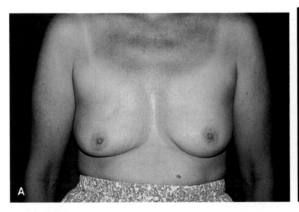 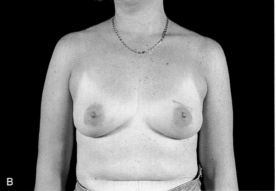

**FIGURE 5-7.**   (**A**) A 2 × 6 cm resection of the right supra-areolar biopsy site, with a radially oriented 3 × 3 × 4 cm parenchymal resection without parenchymal closure. (**B**) After a skin incision nearly parallel to RSTL and a 2 × 2 × 4 cm radial parenchymal resection and parenchymal approximation, there is mild supra-areolar flattening but reasonable breast-shape symmetry.

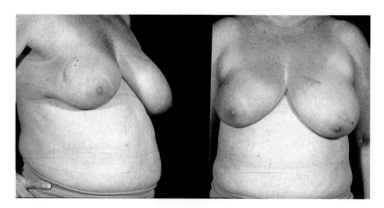

**FIGURE 5-8.** Induration, telangiectasia and upward retraction were noted on this breast 14 months post-radiation. This result was deemed excellent by the patient and radio-therapist. The general surgeon and plastic surgeon defined the outcome as good to fair.

## Reexcision Partial Mastectomy

Reexcision may pose challenging diagnostic and therapeutic dilemmas, particularly when the original biopsy has been performed elsewhere. Usually, a firm biopsy cavity filled with fluid is present after the initial biopsy. When possible, it is desirable to delay reexcision of a large hematoma for 4 to 6 weeks, until the seroma and surrounding inflammatory process lessens or disappears. When this is not possible or when the surgeon unexpectedly enters the biopsy cavity, care should be taken to remove the entire pocket.

When a reexcision is performed after a prior wire localization biopsy, it is vitally important to repeat the mammogram preoperatively. Residual calcifications may require relocalization.

It is useful to use more than one localizing wire to bracket the area in question during reexcision of microcalcifications representing DCIS, particularly when a large area is involved (Fig. 5-9).

If the original resection of breast tissue was large relative to the size of the breast and reexcision is indicated, mastectomy with or without reconstruction is indicated.

## ✦ COMPLICATIONS

After a large resection, significant bleeding may occur. Patients with hematomas that are identified within the first 12 hours should be returned to the operating room for evacuation. Hematomas that develop or are detected later are managed expectantly, with aspiration being clearly indicated if pain, erythema, or impending rupture are noted (Fig. 5-10). Resolution may take as long as 6 or 8 weeks.

Some surgeons believe that the development of a seroma aids in the ultimate cosmetic result. This is a fallacy. The postoperative-volume deficit is temporarily filled by seroma, giving the semblance of an aesthetic repair. An intense, sometimes painful inflammatory response may occur, with significant fibrosis and scar deformity of the skin, parenchyma, or both. If radiation of the wound bed follows (usually within 4 weeks), exaggerated retraction and breast deformity may occur.

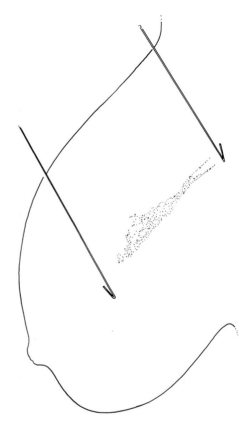

**FIGURE 5-9.** Bracketing.

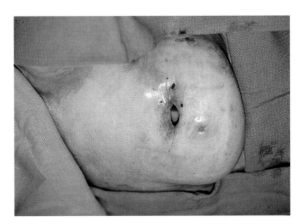

**FIGURE 5-10.** A postoperative seroma ruptured and became infected, delaying radiation therapy for 5 weeks.

**TABLE 5-1**
Patient Survey Results

|  | (n) | (%) |
| --- | --- | --- |
| ***Question: If cancer were to develop in the opposite breast, would you prefer:*** | | |
| Lumpectomy with radiotherapy | 38 | 69 |
| Total mastectomy | 9 | 16 |
| Total mastectomy with breast reconstruction | 9 | 16 |

Seromas are virtually inevitable and many surgeons do not routinely drain or aspirate seromas unless the patient experiences discomfort, the collection threatens rupture, or signs of infection develop (see Fig. 5-10). Serial sterile aspirations lessen patient discomfort and may expedite healing when seromas are very large.

## ◆ PATIENT SATISFACTION WITH AESTHETIC OUTCOME

The interpretation of the cosmetic outcome after partial mastectomy depends on the individual assessing the outcome. The surgeon and oncologist view the partial mastectomy deformity by comparing the operated and normal breasts, whereas the patient compares what may even be a deformed breast to the alternative of no breast at all.

Functional and cosmetic deformities after breast conservation may become notable long after the operation because all patients develop some edema and fibrosis that lasts for 12 to 48 months. Telangiectasia develops in 24 to 48 months and is virtually always persistent.

Despite these considerations, when a patient who has undergone breast conservation is questioned regarding whether the same therapy would be chosen if a contralateral cancer developed, more than 70% answer in the affirmative (Table 5-1).[8]

## REFERENCES

1. Veronesi U, Banfi A, Del Vecchio M, et al. Comparison of Halsted mastectomy with quandrentectomy, axillary dissection and radiotherapy in early breast cancer: long-term results. Eur J Cancer Clin Oncol 1986;22:1085.
2. Schnitt SJ, Connolly JL. Processing and evaluation of breast excision specimens. A clinically oriented approach. Anat Pathol 1992;98:126.
3. Boyages J, Recht A, Connolly J, et al. Early breast cancer: predictors of breast recurrence for patients treated with conservative surgery and radiation therapy. Radiother Oncol 1990;19:29.
4. Holland R, Connolly Gelman R, et al. The presence of an extensive intraductal component (EIC) following a limited excision correlates with prominent residual disease in the remainder of the breast. J Clin Oncol 1990;8:113.

5. Calle R, Viloq JR, Zafrani B. Local control and survival of breast cancer treated by limited surgery followed by irradiation. Int J Radiol Oncol Biophys 1986;12:873.

6. Lindley R, Bulman A, Parson P, et al. Histological features predictive of an increased risk of early local recurrence after treatment of breast cancer by local tumor excision and radical radiotherapy. Surgery 1989;105:13.

7. Schnitt SJ, Abner A, Gelman R, et al. The relationship between microscopic margins of resection and the risk of local recurrence in patients with breast cancer treated with breast conserving surgery and radiation therapy. Cancer 1994;74:1476.

8. Matory WE Jr, Wertheimer M, Fitzgerald TJ, et al. Aesthetic results following partial mastectomy and radiation. Plast Reconstr Surg 1990;85:739.

9. Matory WE Jr, Wertheimer M, Love S. Optimizing aesthetics following partial mastectomy. Breast Dis 1992;5:225.

10. Lagios M, Gates B, Zestdahl PR, et al. A guide to the frequency of nipple involvement in breast cancer. Am J Surg 1979;138:135.

*Atlas of Techniques in Breast Surgery,*
by William Silen, W. Earle Matory, Jr. and Susan M. Love.
Lippincott-Raven Publishers, Philadelphia, © 1996.

# Chapter 6

# Axillary Dissection

T he goals of axillary dissections are to (1) stage for prognostic purposes, (2) prevent axillary recurrence, and (3) in some instances influence the use of adjuvant therapy. The study of extended radical mastectomy by Veronesi and Valagussa[1] and the National Surgical Adjuvant Breast Protocol (NSABP) study[2] that compared total mastectomy with or without radiation therapy with modified radical mastectomy both showed that extensive nodal resection does not enhance survival. Several studies, however, have helped to define the extent of axillary dissection necessary to achieve the above goals (Fig. 6-1).[3–6] Steele and coworkers found that removal of at least four axillary nodes (usually in level I of the axilla) provides adequate staging and that skip nodal lesions involving level III are rare (about 4%) in the absence of level I involvement.[3] Other studies have supported the finding that even relatively small axillary dissections (six nodes or more) may provide protection against future axillary recurrence, thus averting the need for radiation of the axilla.[2,4,7]

The NSABP B-04 study,[2] Cancer Research Campaign (CRC) Working Party,[8] and Manchester[9] studies demonstrated that primary treatment of the axillary nodes had no impact on long-term survival. The NSABP B-04[2] and CRC trials[8] showed that waiting to treat axillary nodes by excision or radiation therapy until the appearance of gross disease rather than prophylactically had no adverse impact on long-term survival. Thus initial axillary dissection is directed primarily at determining prognosis and only secondarily for local control.

Although few would argue with axillary sampling to determine prognosis, its use for identifying those women who will benefit from adjuvant therapy is in question. At least 20% of women with uninvolved axillary nodes by conventional pathologic evaluation can be found to have micrometastases in the axillary nodes if serial sections are examined. At least 30% of women with negative axillary nodes have a systemic recurrence. Other biologic markers such as tumor size, number of blood vessels, vas-

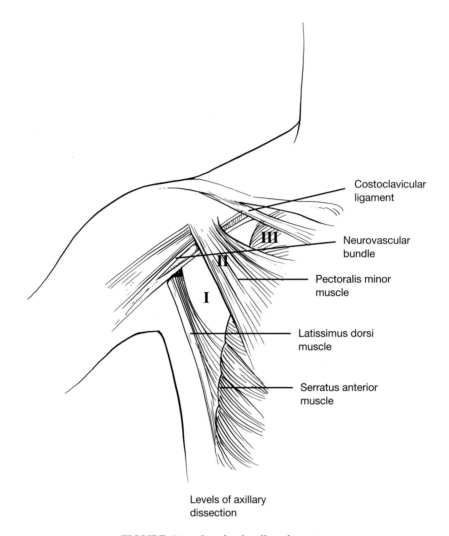

Costoclavicular
ligament

Neurovascular
bundle

Pectoralis minor
muscle

Latissimus dorsi
muscle

Serratus anterior
muscle

Levels of axillary
dissection

**FIGURE 6-1.** Levels of axillary dissection.

cular invasion, ploidy, S-phase, Her-2-*neu* oncogene overexpression, cathepsin D, or heat-shock protein may prove useful in identifying these women. The increasing use of adjuvant systemic therapy for almost all women having breast cancer, regardless of nodal status, also raises the question of the need for axillary surgery.

At this time we believe that there is no better prognostic indicator than the status of the axillary nodes. An alternative to using axillary dissection as an aid in deciding for or against adjuvant therapy is to treat all women with systemic chemotherapy. This approach has been suggested, most notably, for the use of tamoxifen in older women. Tamoxifen, however, is not without toxicity, as illustrated by the deaths of six women from tamoxifen-induced uterine cancer in the NSABP B-14 study.[10] In addition, tamoxifen is expensive and may be associated with significant side effects. The finding of uninvolved nodes in a woman with other good prognostic indicators could eliminate the need for years of adjuvant tamoxifen therapy. For this reason, an axillary dissection may have its most significant clinical import in women having small tumors.

Although regional recurrence does not adversely affect survival, patients experience considerable distress at the time of tumor recurrence. For this reason, we believe that axillary nodes should either be dissected or irradiated at the time of the initial definitive treatment. The minimum number of nodes that must be removed to prevent local recurrence is suggested by the results of several studies. NSABP study B-04[2] indicates that six nodes confer protection, whereas studies from Edinburgh[3] and Kjaergaard and coworkers[4] suggest that even removal of only three or four may be protective. A complete level I dissection is termed a lateral axillary dissection by some.

Although it is possible that in the future axillary dissection may be abandoned, the preponderance of opinion at this time is that at least a level I or combined level I and II dissection is indicated in most women having invasive breast cancer. The dissection is best defined anatomically, rather than by the number of nodes that have been removed.

Axillary dissection is similar, whether it is performed as part of a modified radical–total mastectomy, partial mastectomy, or an isolated procedure. At the time of total mastectomy, the axillary dissection is usually in continuity with the breast resection. With partial mastectomy, the axillary dissection is preferably not in continuity unless the primary lesion is in the tail of the breast; is small, requiring minimal resection of breast volume; and is within 4 to 5 cm of the anterior axillary line (Figs. 6-2 and 6-3).

## ✦ OPERATIVE TECHNIQUE

The patient is positioned supine on the operating table, with the arm at a right angle to the trunk. Some surgeons place a pillow or folded towel under the scapula to hyperabduct the shoulder.

A skin marker is used to outline the edge of the pectoralis major and the latissimus dorsi. If the procedure is to be performed through a separate incision, a transverse incision that courses within resting skin tension lines is preferred to those that are oblique or vertical, which may lead to contracture. The incision placed just be-

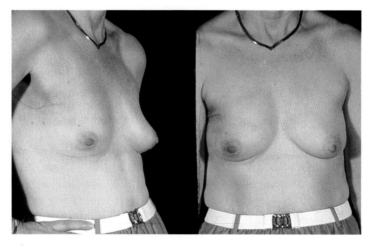

**FIGURE 6-2.**    An in-continuity resection of a primary lesion in the far upper-outer quadrant of the breast combined with an axillary dissection, with reasonable aesthetic outcome.

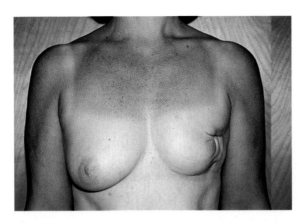

**FIGURE 6-3.** Suboptimal cosmesis following a combined excision of the primary lesion with an axillary dissection, very likely due to the tumor's location over 4 cm from the axillary dissection.

low the axillary hairline (Fig. 6-4*A*) extends from just posterior to the sulcus along the lateral border of the pectoralis major to the depression just anterior to the latissimus dorsi. If the incision extends further onto the border of the either muscle, scars will be visible when a sleeveless dress is worn.

The incision is carried through the dermis and fat with electrocautery. On identification of the axillary fascia, it is incised (see Fig. 6-4*B*), revealing the axillary fat pad (see Fig. 6-4*C*). A Wheatlander self-retaining retractor is used to spread the wound edges. The lateral border of the pectoralis major muscle is identified and cleared. Blunt and sharp dissection with a Metzenbaum scissor or with a right-angled clamp provides ideal exposure.

The medial pectoral nerve branches to the pectoralis major are identified and preserved. The dissection is continued deep to the pectoralis major, sweeping Rotter's interpectoral nodes laterally. A retractor is placed under the pectoralis major and minor (a fiberoptic lighted right-angle–Florence Nightingale retractor optimizes exposure) and the adipose tissue is swept laterally from the undersurface of the pectoralis minor, thus clearing level II nodes up to the medial border of the pectoralis minor (see Fig. 6-4*B* through *E*).

The axillary vein is identified at the superior extent of the wound. The adventitia of the axillary vein is preserved because resection provides no therapeutic or diagnostic benefit. In addition, stripping of the adventitia may promote thrombosis, which contributes to the development of chronic upper extremity edema. The axillary fat is swept inferiorly from the vein and laterally from the chest wall. The intercostobrachiocutaneous nerve is identified as it emerges from the serratus anterior muscle and courses into the axillary fat pad toward the upper inner arm. The nerve is carefully dissected by opening the fat pad and tracing the nerve through the axillary fat. The specimen can be removed in two segments if this is helpful in preserving the nerve.

As the dissection continues inferiorly and laterally, the long thoracic nerve (Fig. 6-4*D*) is identified and preserved as it descends vertically along the chest wall to innervate the serratus anterior muscle. The axillary fat pad is dissected from lateral to medial along the latissimus dorsi after identifying and preserving the thoracodorsal nerve, artery, and vein. Often a second intercostal sensory branch crosses the axilla; it too is preserved. Once the thoracodorsal and long thoracic nerves have been identified, the axillary pad lying between them on the subscapular muscle is dissected caudally to the tail of the breast (see Fig. 6-4*D* and *E*). We do not use clips nor do we

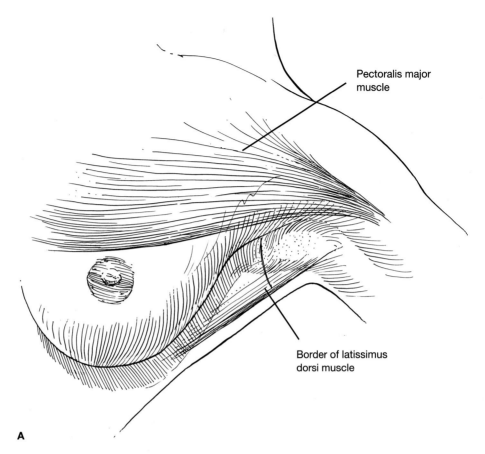

Pectoralis major
muscle

Border of latissimus
dorsi muscle

**A**

**FIGURE 6-4.** **(A)** Skin incision. **(B)** Opening of the axillary fascia and identification of the pectoralis major muscle anteriorly and the latissimus dorsi muscle posteriorly. **(C)** Identification of the axillary vein and dissection of the tissue inferiorly. **(D)** Dissection of the tissue between the long thoracic nerve and the thoracodorsal nerve. **(E)** Completed dissection.

ligate lymphatic branches. After hemostasis is achieved, 10 mL of 0.5% bupivacaine is instilled into the wound to mitigate postoperative pain.

## ✦ LEVEL III DISSECTION

Some surgeons routinely include level III in every axillary dissection. As discussed above, there is no evidence that inclusion of level III reduces the incidence of subsequent axillary recurrence. It is possible that the incidence of postoperative edema may be increased by this procedure, and the maximum failure to stage the disease properly by omission of level III is no more than 4%. For these reasons, we usually carry out a combined level I and II dissection only. If the surgeon chooses to include level III, the pectoralis major muscle is identified and dissected as described. The lymphatic and fatty tissue under the pectoralis major muscle is dissected and the coracobrachial fascia is incised from the coracobrachial muscle toward the insertion

*(text continues on p. 82)*

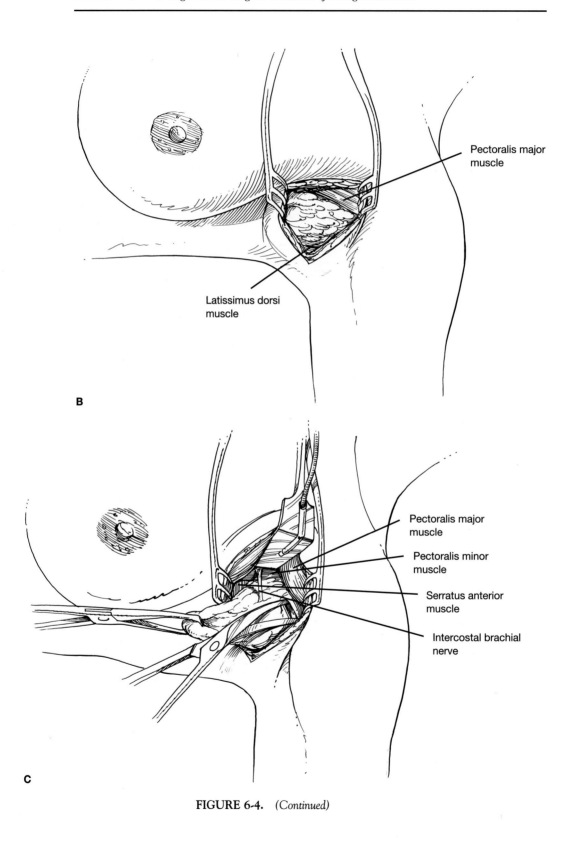

Pectoralis major
muscle

Latissimus dorsi
muscle

**B**

Pectoralis major
muscle

Pectoralis minor
muscle

Serratus anterior
muscle

Intercostal brachial
nerve

**C**

**FIGURE 6-4.** *(Continued)*

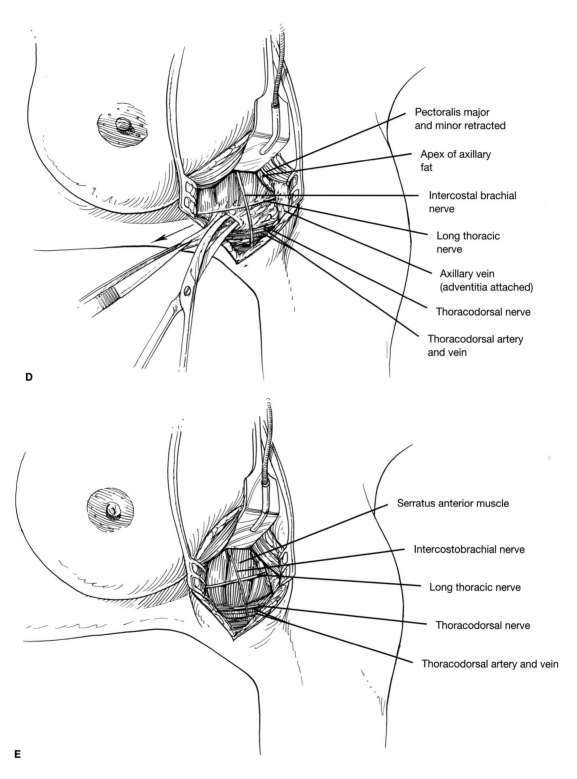

**D**

Pectoralis major
and minor retracted

Apex of axillary
fat

Intercostal brachial
nerve

Long thoracic
nerve

Axillary vein
(adventitia attached)

Thoracodorsal nerve

Thoracodorsal artery
and vein

**E**

Serratus anterior muscle

Intercostobrachial nerve

Long thoracic nerve

Thoracodorsal nerve

Thoracodorsal artery and vein

**FIGURE 6-4.**  *(Continued)*

of the pectoralis minor. The pectoralis minor muscle is divided at its insertion and allowed to retract inferiorly. This permits exposure of the axillary vein medially as it crosses beneath the costoclavicular ligament. The long thoracic and thoracodorsal nerves are identified and preserved. All the fat and axillary tissue is then exposed laterally and the pectoralis minor muscle may be removed with the axillary specimen, or it may be left attached to the chest wall. The intercostal brachial nerve and the third intercostal nerve are sometimes sacrificed if these structures significantly interfere with the dissection. The dissection proceeds laterally in the manner that was previously described.

## ✦ DRAINAGE OF THE AXILLA

The decision to drain the axilla is based on surgeon preference. A growing number of surgeons choose not to drain the axilla because of the relatively low incidence of symptomatic seroma, even though some prospective trials have shown that drainage decreases this problem, especially when motion of the shoulder is limited.[11,12] The development of a large axillary seroma, however, can be highly problematic because of pain, subsequent infection, or postradiation retraction. When immediate breast reconstruction is performed, drainage is preferred to minimize periprosthetic or subflap seroma formation.

## ✦ POSTOPERATIVE CARE

Controversy exists regarding the amount of mobility that should be allowed postoperatively. Several proper randomized trials have shown that delaying motion of the shoulder, especially abduction, reduces the incidence of complications due to elevation of skin flaps, which often results in chronic seroma or subsequent infection without an increase in the incidence of frozen shoulders.[11-13] Early active motion increases the accumulation of seroma fluid.

One important measure to reduce troublesome secondary complications of seroma is the careful approximation of axillary fascia. The deep dermis is also brought together with absorbable suture and the skin is closed with a subcuticular suture, with steristrips applied to the skin.

## ✦ COMPLICATIONS

Common concerns after axillary dissection include injury to the intercostobrachial nerve and its branches. This preventable event causes considerable symptomatology due to numbness of the posterior aspect of the axilla and the upper inner arm. A winged scapula due to palsy of the serratus anterior muscle secondary to injury of the long thoracic nerve has been reported in 10% of patients after axillary dissection. Winging is often temporary, usually resolving in 6 weeks to 6 months (see Fig. 1-15).

Axillary vein phlebitis is more common when the vein is stripped of its adventitia. Because the goals of axillary dissection do not warrant this maneuver, one is advised to avoid stripping. In addition, phlebitis is probably less likely if direct tributaries of the axillary vein are ligated flush with the main vessel.

Lymph fistula is not as common as feared. In a series of 250 lateral axillary dissections treated without postoperative drains, aspiration of seromas was deemed necessary only 10% of the time.[14] This may be attributable to careful closure of the axillary fascia. Delayed arm mobilization may further limit seroma formation.[11–13] In contrast, frozen shoulder is a function of prolonged immobility. Stiffness can be avoided with rigorous physical therapy beginning 10 to 12 days after surgery.

Immediate breast reconstruction imposes additional concerns based on the problematic ramifications of periprosthetic or subflap seromas. After latissimus flap reconstruction, patients should be mobilized early to prevent shoulder contracture and also require drains to the back, chest, and axilla.

One of the most serious and debilitating postoperative sequelae is lymphedema. The more extensive the axillary dissection, the greater risk. When axillary radiation is added to removal of axillary nodes, the risk of lymphedema is markedly increased. Chronic lymphedema is often a late sequela, developing 12 to 36 months or more after axillary dissection. Patients should be questioned about inability to wear rings or watches, poor clothing fit, arm pain and swelling, carpal tunnel or other compression neuropathies, and recurrent infections. Lymphedema, if treated as soon as it develops, often responds well to short- or long-term use of pneumatic compression devices that are used at home for 2 to 8 hours daily. The more chronic type of lymphedema is more resistant to therapy.

### REFERENCES

1. Veronesi U, Valagussa P. Ineffecacy of internal mammary node dissection in breast cancer surgery. Cancer 1981;47:170.
2. Fisher B, Redmond C, Fisher E, et al. Ten year results of a randomized clinical trial comparing radical mastectomy and total mastectomy with and without radiation. N Engl J Med 1985;312:674.
3. Steele RJC, Forrest APM, Gibson T, et al. The efficacy of lower axillary sampling in obtaining lymph node status in breast cancer: a controlled randomized trial. Br J Surg 1985;72:368.
4. Kjaergaard J, Blichert-Toft M, Andersen JA, et al. Probability of false negative nodal staging in conjunction with partial axillary dissection in breast cancer. Br J Surg 1985;72:365.
5. Pigott J, Nichols J, Maddox WA, et al. Metastases to the upper levels of the axillary nodes in carcinoma of the breast and its implications for nodal sampling procedures. Surg Gynecol Obstet 1984;158:225.
6. Veronesi U, Luini A, Galimberti V, et al. Extent of metastatic axillary involvement in 1446 cases of breast cancer. Eur J Surg Oncol 1990;16:127.
7. Dewar JA, Sarrazin D, Benhamou S, et al. Management of the axilla in conservatively treated breast cancer 592 patients treated at Institut Gustave-Roussy. Int J Radiat Oncol Biol Phys 1987;13:475.
8. Cancer Research Campaign Working Party. Cancer research campaign (King's/Cambridge) trial for early breast cancer. Lancet 1980;2:55.
9. Lythgoe JP, Palmer MK. Manchester regional breast study: five and ten year results. Br J Surg 1982;69:693.
10. Fisher B. Tamoxifen for the treatment of node negative breast cancer patients with estrogen receptor positive tumors: results from NSABP protocol B14. N Engl J Med 1989;320:479.
11. Dawson I, Stam I, Heslinga JM. Effect of shoulder immobilization on wound seroma and

shoulder dysfunction following radical mastectomy. A randomized prospective clinical trial. Br J Surg 1989;76:311.

12. Flew TJ. Wound drainage following radical mastectomy. The effect of restriction of shoulder movement. Br J Surg 1979;66:302.

13. Lotze MT, Duncan MA, Gerberg LH, et al. Early versus delayed shoulder motion following axillary dissection. Ann Surg 1981;193:288.

14. Siegel BM, Mayzel KH, Love SM. Level I and II axillary dissection in the treatment of early stage breast cancer; an analysis of 259 consecutive patients. Arch Surg 1990; 125:1144.

*Atlas of Techniques in Breast Surgery,*
by William Silen, W. Earle Matory, Jr. and Susan M. Love.
Lippincott-Raven Publishers, Philadelphia, © 1996.

*Chapter* 7

# Total Mastectomy (Modified Radical Mastectomy)

The techniques of total or modified radical mastectomy vary from one surgeon to another. As one author (W. Silen) is fond of saying, "they call it a modified radical mastectomy because everyone has his or her own modification." When Halsted developed the radical mastectomy in 1882, local control was a major challenge because cancers were extensive and it was necessary to resect large segments of skin and muscle to encompass the gross tumor. Before the development of effective radiation and chemotherapy, the Halsted radical mastectomy became the standard technique because it seemed logical that the disease progressed sequentially from a localized primary lesion to the regional lymph nodes and only subsequently to the blood stream. Not only was it considered mandatory to remove all of the breast tissue but it was deemed critical to excise large margins of skin, develop very thin skin flaps, dissect all three levels of the axilla, and resect both pectoral muscles. In the 1960s and even earlier, some adventuresome surgeons (Patey) began to reduce the extent of the classic Halsted radical mastectomy, developing a procedure that approximates the contemporary modified radical mastectomy.[1] Subsequent controlled trials indicate that the radical mastectomy is not superior to modified radical mastectomy in terms of survival;[2,3] therefore, the classic Halsted radical mastectomy has become virtually obsolete.

It has been estimated that only 30% of women with early breast cancer require a mastectomy for local control; the remainder are candidates for breast conservation. Despite this, most women in the United States continue to undergo mastectomy as primary treatment. The prime indication for mastectomy is clear: a tumor that is too large to remove without producing significant cosmetic deformity. Mastectomy is thus performed in cases of relatively large (T3) lesions for locally advanced disease that has not become downstaged after neoadjuvant chemotherapy and in instances of extensive intraductal carcinoma. Another common indication is patient or physician preference, often influenced strongly by prejudice and the fear of or difficulties of long-term surveillance.

Total mastectomy is the preferable nomenclature for a surgical procedure designed to remove all of the mammary tissue. The terms simple and total mastectomy are often used interchangeably but because simple mastectomy implies to some removal of only the protuberant portion of the breast, the two procedures should be clearly distinguished from each other. The term modified radical mastectomy does not specify the extent of axillary dissection. It is undoubtedly more precise to refer to the modified radical mastectomy as a mastectomy while also indicating the specific level (I, II, or III) of the axillary dissection (see Fig. 6-1).

## ✦ OPERATIVE TECHNIQUE: SKIN INCISIONS, SKIN-PRESERVING INCISIONS

The purpose of resection of skin as a component of mastectomy is to remove the potentially tumor-bearing skin. At the same time, an aesthetic scar that is free of redundant skin should also be achieved. These goals are best achieved by excision of an ellipse of skin. When immediate reconstruction is contemplated, a skin-sparing or "jigsaw" pattern can be employed (Fig. 7-1*A* through *L*).

The ellipse is preferably oriented horizontally to minimize visibility of the resultant scar (Fig. 7-1*A, C,* and *D*). The biopsy site and nipple–areolar complex are excised with a margin of as little as 1 cm, depending on the position of the biopsy site. The incision should be along resting skin tension lines and extended far enough medially and laterally to avoid redundant skin at each end (dog ears). Breast parenchyma extends superiorly to the clavicle, medially to the sternum, laterally to the latissimus dorsi, and inferiorly toward the costal margin (3 to 4 cm below the inframammary fold; Fig. 7-2*A*). The design of the skin flaps should therefore provide sufficient access to excise all breast tissue. Before incision, it is advisable to mark on the skin the proposed elliptical cutaneous excision and the proposed extent of the excision of mammary tissue to avoid making the skin flaps excessively long.

If an axillary dissection is to be included, its extent should be planned preoperatively. Our preference is to dissect levels I and II of the axilla but some surgeons continue to remove nodes from all three levels.

The skin incision is made with a sharp blade, which is then exchanged for the electrocautery. The latter is used to incise the dermis and to develop the skin flaps and for most of the mastectomy, although equally good results can be obtained with a cold scalpel in a feathering style and or with the $CO_2$ laser. Skin hooks are placed in the superior flap at its cut edge and traction is exerted by an assistant in a direction perpendicular to the chest wall (Fig. 7-2*B*). The surgeon maintains countertraction on the breast using the nondominant hand, making the plane between breast parenchyma and subcutaneous fat more apparent. Thin flaps including dermis and a 1-cm layer of subcutaneous fat are made using the electrocautery, with care taken to avoid making a buttonhole in the flap (Fig. 7-2*C*). As the level of the clavicle is approached, the dissection is gradually deepened to the fibers of the pectoralis major. Skin flaps are developed in a similar manner medi-

*(text continues on p. 93)*

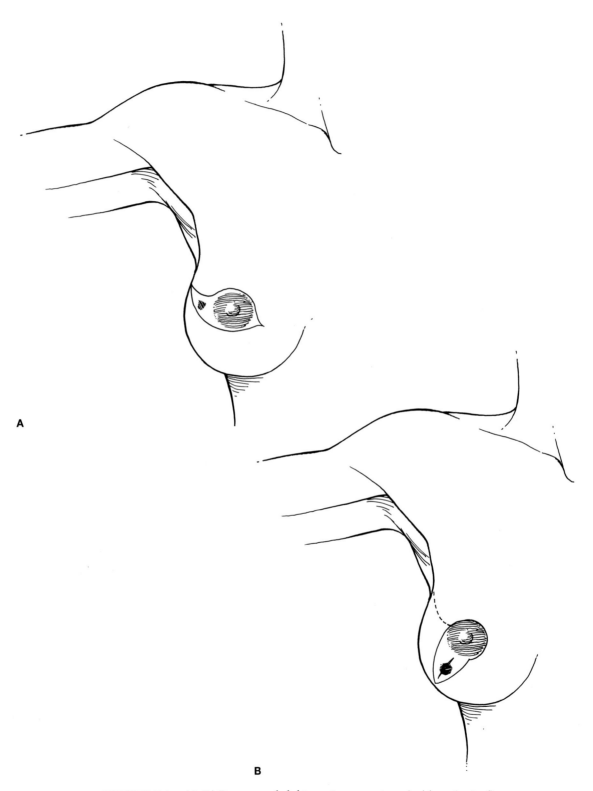

**FIGURE 7-1.**   (A–L) Recommended skin-saving mastectomy incisions. (*continued*)

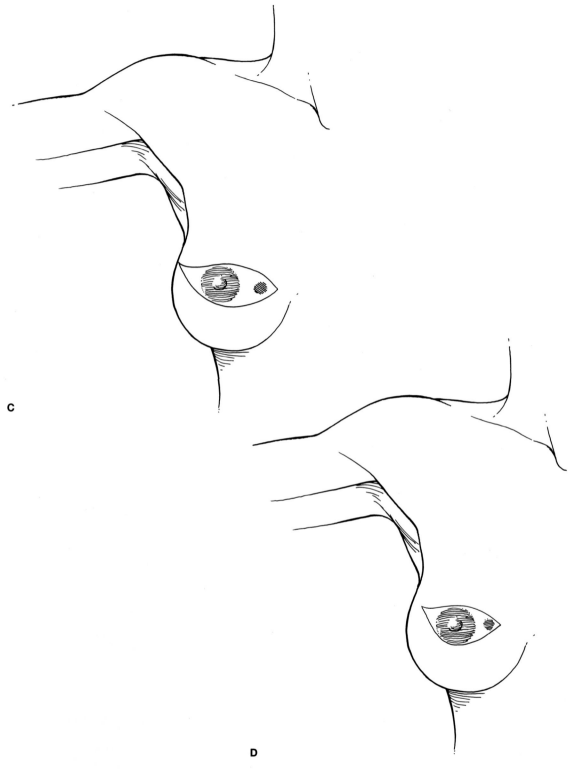

C

D

**FIGURE 7-1.**   *(Continued)*

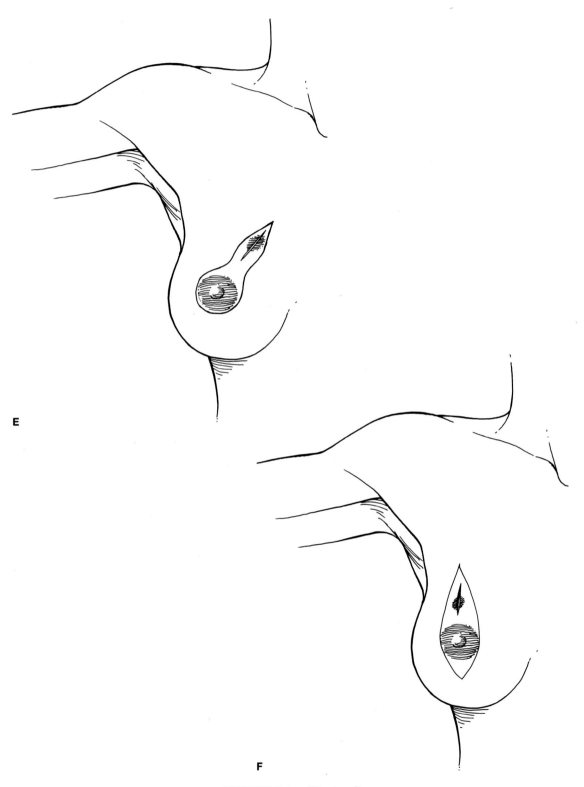

E

F

**FIGURE 7-1.** *(Continued)*

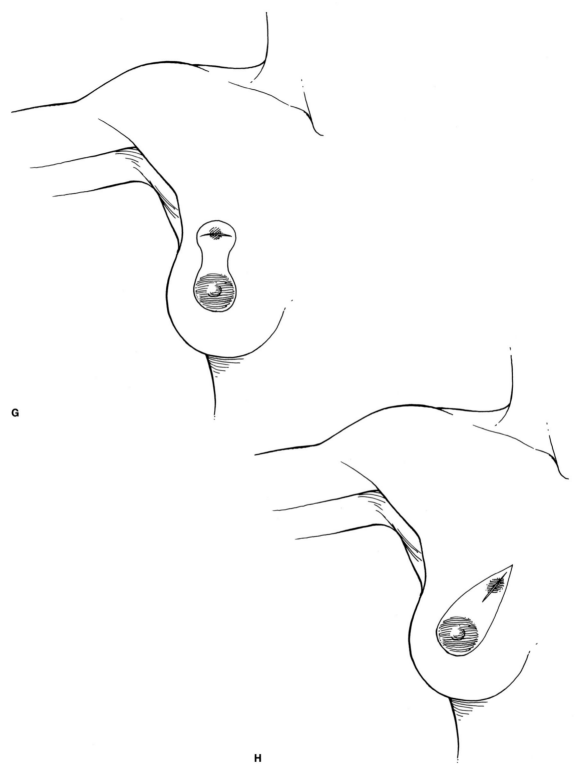

G

H

**FIGURE 7-1.** *(Continued)*

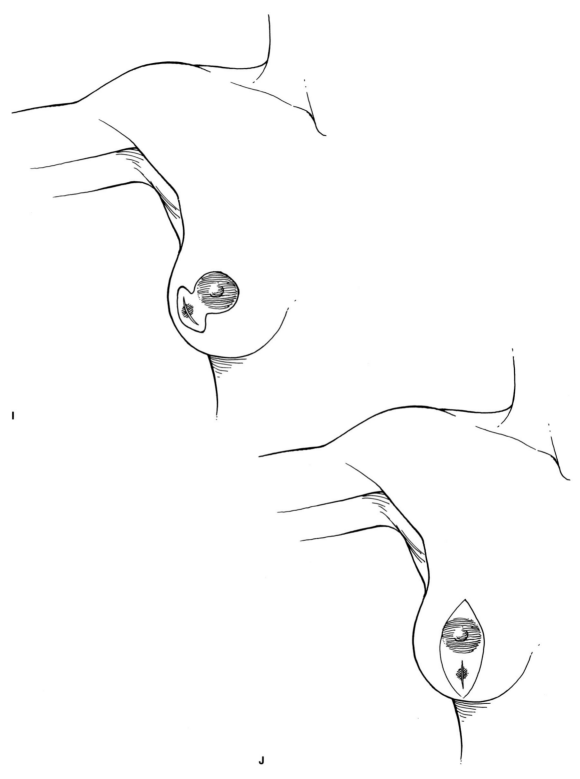

**FIGURE 7-1.** *(Continued)*

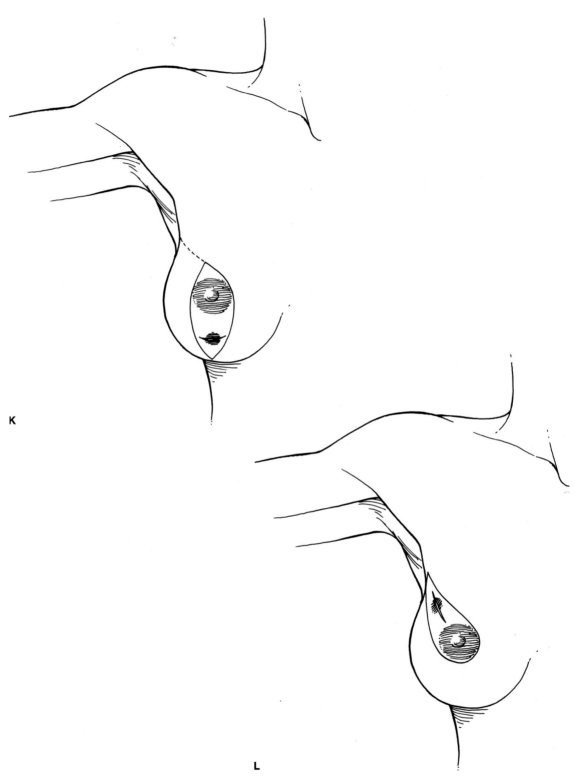

K

L

**FIGURE 7-1.** *(Continued)*

ally to the lateral border of the sternum, inferiorly 2 to 3 cm below the inframammary fold, and laterally to the anterior border of the latissimus dorsi muscle. The breast is dissected from the pectoralis major muscle medially, taking care to include the pectoralis fascia with the specimen. The intercostal perforators of the internal mammary artery are ligated or suture-ligated with 3-0 absorbable suture (Fig. 7-2*E*). It is important to prevent retraction of these vessels through the intercostal muscles into the chest cavity. Searching for them may lead to an inadvertent pneumothorax. The dissection is then continued from medial to lateral. The dissection plane becomes easier as Cooper's ligaments of the breast begin to disappear toward the lateral border of the pectoralis major (Fig. 7-2*E* and *F*). The weight of the breast is allowed to exert traction laterally, and the axillary fascia is identified as it encompasses the pectoralis minor (Fig. 7-34*G*). The axillary fascia is carefully incised, watching for and preserving the branches of the medial pectoral nerve and the lateral thoracic artery and vein as they pass around and through the pectoralis minor to enter the deep surface of the pectoralis major. Injury to the medial pectoral nerve results in atrophy of the lower third to half of the pectoralis muscle and may lead to significant chest wall deformity. The nodes lying between the pectoralis major and minor are swept laterally and a retractor is placed under the two muscles to facilitate dissection along the axillary vein, if such is to be carried out.

If the axilla is not to be dissected, attention is shifted to completion of the lateral portion of the mastectomy. Care must be taken to avoid dissecting between the interdigitations of the serratus but this is more likely to occur if the dissection on the chest wall at this point is carried from medial to lateral. Dissection the breast from the serratus anterior muscle is best performed by proceeding from lateral to medial. The anterolateral border of the latissimus dorsi muscle is identified and the fibrofatty tissue along its border is swept medially with the specimen (Fig. 7-2*D*).

The resected specimen is oriented for the pathologist by placing marking sutures in the axilla and at twelve o'clock on the skin. The specimen is sent fresh, so that estrogen receptors and any other tests (flow cytometry) can be obtained. The pathologist should ink the deep margin before breadloafing the specimen to enable a better evaluation of the deep margin histologically. Although we believe that it is probably important to assess the presence or absence of involvement of the deep margin, at least one study has shown no relation between involvement of the deep margin and the incidence of subsequent local recurrence.[4]

The mastectomy site is then irrigated using saline, and meticulous attention is given to achieving excellent hemostasis. Suction drains are placed in the axilla (taking care to avoid placing the drain on the intercostal brachial nerve or on the axillary vein) and across the lower anterior chest. The drains are brought out through separate stab wounds (preferably hidden in the axilla) and are sutured in place. The skin–fat flaps are inspected to ensure that they will approximate without undue tension and without dog ears. To avoid the latter in the ptotic or large-breasted patient, additional skin may need to be resected laterally or a lateral V-shaped wedge can be created to eliminate the excess skin (Fig. 7-2*H*). This obviates the problem of a large tag of skin and fat in the axilla that hangs over the bra and rubs against the medial axilla, a source of constant irritation for many women. The subcutaneous fat is closed with 3-0 interrupted absorbable suture and skin is ap-

*(text continues on p. 96)*

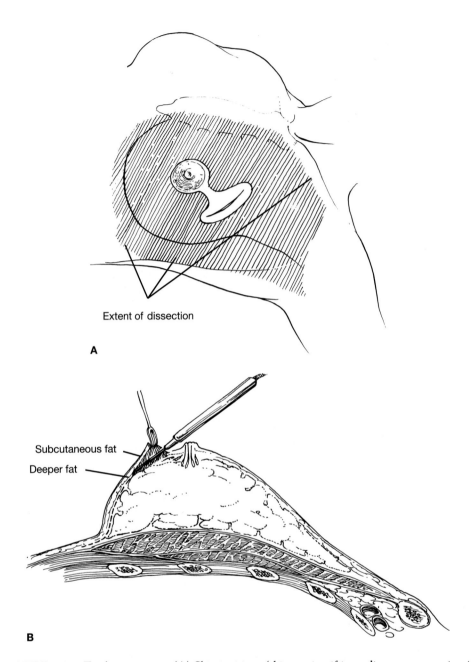

Extent of dissection

**A**

Subcutaneous fat

Deeper fat

**B**

**FIGURE 7-2.**   Total mastectomy. (**A**) Skin incisions (skin-sparing if immediate reconstruction is contemplated). (**A and B**) Developing the skin flaps and extent of the resection. (**C**) Completion of skin flaps. (**D**) Identification of the lateral border of latissimus dorsi muscle. (**E**) Subfascial dissection and ligation of internal mammary perforators. (**F**) Lateral dissection of breast from chest wall. (**G**) Beginning of axillary dissection. (**H**) Closing skin with attention to the lateral dog ear. (**I**) Drains and steristrips. (**J**) Dressing.

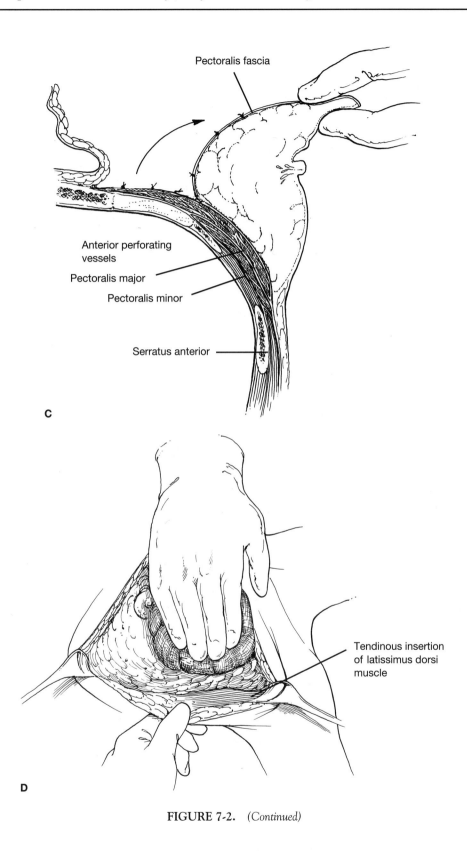

FIGURE 7-2.  *(Continued)*

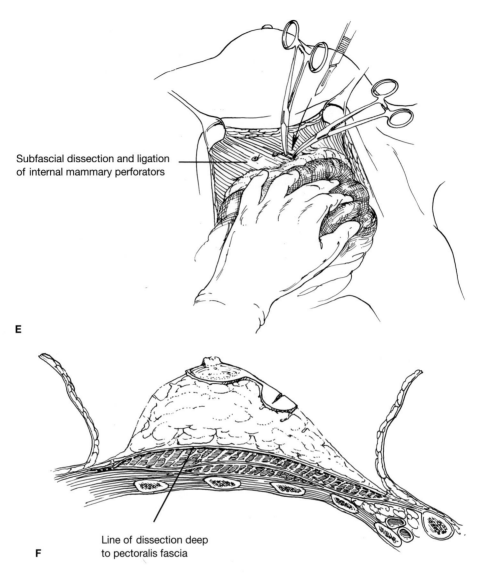

Subfascial dissection and ligation
of internal mammary perforators

E

Line of dissection deep
to pectoralis fascia

F

**FIGURE 7-2.** *(Continued)*

proximated with an absorbable running subcuticular stitch. Although other methods of skin closure are acceptable, this technique avoids the need for suture removal, which may prove to be somewhat uncomfortable along the postoperative dysesthetic mastectomy incision.

A bulky dressing is applied and loosely taped with one piece of tape (Fig. 7-2*J*). A bias-cut stockinet is wrapped around the trunk of the patient and over the shoulder to encompass the bulky dressings and both breasts. This minimizes the amount of tape needed, while giving the patient an element of protection. A sling or sling and swath are optional.

The drain reservoirs are emptied every 8 hours and are removed when there is less than 30 mL/24 hours or at 4 or 5 days, whichever comes first. The patient may

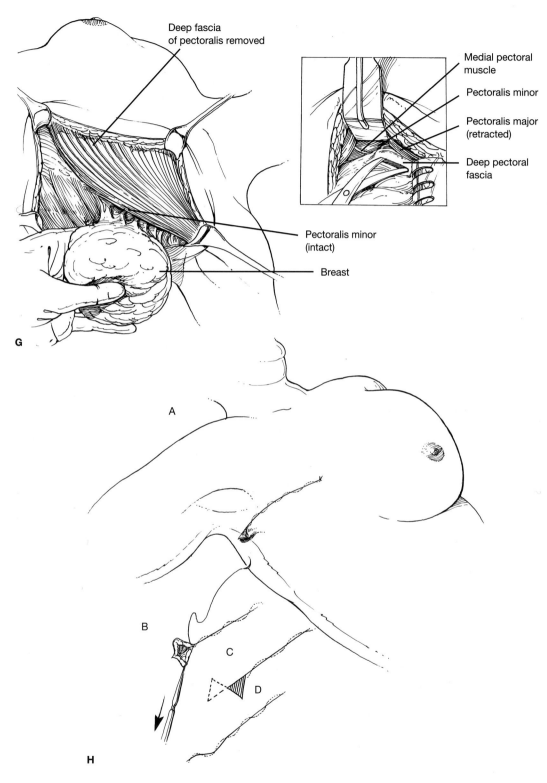

Deep fascia
of pectoralis removed

Medial pectoral
muscle

Pectoralis minor

Pectoralis major
(retracted)

Deep pectoral
fascia

Pectoralis minor
(intact)

Breast

G

A

B

C

D

H

**FIGURE 7-2.** *(Continued)*

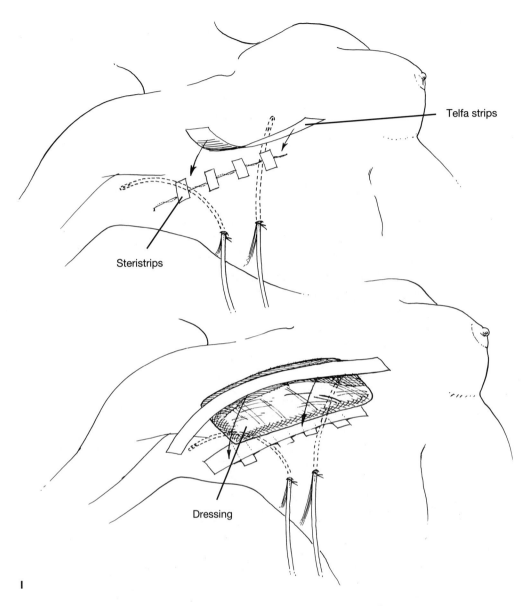

Telfa strips

Steristrips

Dressing

**FIGURE 7-2.**  *(Continued)*

be discharged with the drains in place. The average length of stay is 2 days or less. In many instances, mastectomy without reconstruction can be performed on an outpatient basis.

## ✦ COMPLICATIONS

Postoperative seroma, the most common complication after mastectomy, can be treated by aspiration in the office or may be left to resorb. Aspiration is indicated

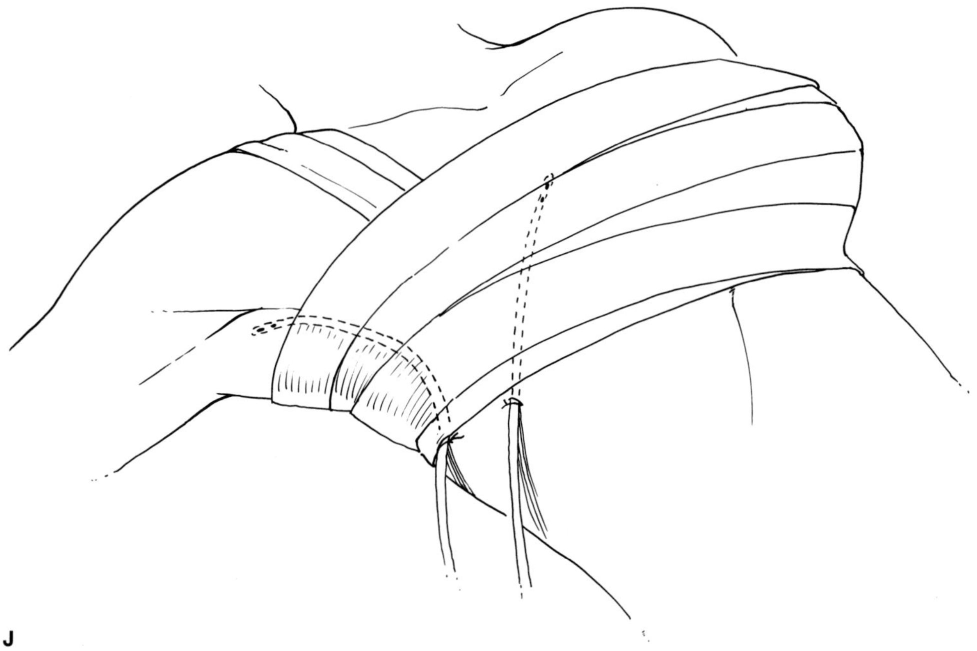

**J**

**FIGURE 7-2.** *(Continued)*

when the seroma threatens viability of the skin flaps, is under tension, or is associated with signs of infection such as fever or cellulitis. Partial necrosis of skin flaps may occur, most commonly as necrosis along the edge of the suture line. This seldom requires debridement. If a larger area of necrosis develops, a wet eschar or infection may supervene, thus requiring debridement and healing by secondary intention.

Without question, mastectomy of any type is a mutilating procedure. A less than aesthetic scar adds additional psychological embarrassment. Dog ears or a poor scar may be modified secondarily under local anesthesia. Many women do not seek reconstruction but desire a neat surgical scar.

Retained breast tissue may lead to recurrence of the malignancy or to the development of a new primary lesion. Thick skin–fat flaps often leave residual glandular tissue in the patient. Whether this makes an overall difference in long-term survival is not clear.

### REFERENCES

1. Patey DH, Dyson WH. The prognosis of carcinoma of the breast in relation to the type of operation performed. Br J Cancer 1948;2:7.
2. Turner L, Swindell R, Bell WGT, et al. Radical versus modified radical mastectomy for breast cancer. Ann R Coll Surg Engl 1981;63:239.
3. Maddox WA, Carpenter JT Jr, Laws HT, et al. A randomized prospective trial of radical (Halsted) mastectomy versus modified radical mastectomy in 311 breast cancer patients. Ann Surg 1983;198:207.
4. Mentzer SJ, Osteen RT, Wilson RE. Local recurrence and the deep resection margin in carcinoma of the breast. Surg Gynecol and Obstet 1986;163:513.

*Atlas of Techniques in Breast Surgery,*
by William Silen, W. Earle Matory, Jr. and Susan M. Love.
Lippincott-Raven Publishers, Philadelphia, © 1996.

# *Chapter* 8

# Radical Mastectomy

There are currently few indications for a radical mastectomy. Large tumors that are fixed to the underlying muscle are usually treated initially with systemic therapy and are thus rendered operable by less-than-radical mastectomy. Rarely, a large tumor fixed to the muscle may require a palliative radical mastectomy. Recurrences that involve the pectoralis muscle or its fascia after local excision and radiation may necessitate radical removal of breast parenchyma and chest wall musculature. It is for these rare occurrences that the following description is included.

## ✦ OPERATIVE TECHNIQUE

The patient should be draped to allow access to an area for a split-thickness skin graft (e.g., the thigh) or for an alternative reconstruction. Skin-graft coverage is far from ideal in most of the circumstances that require radical mastectomy. Vascularized soft-tissue reconstructions with pedicled or free latissimus dorsi or rectus abdominis muscle are preferable to a free skin graft (positioning would then be as described for each specific type of immediate reconstruction). The latter techniques have the advantage of bringing in fresh blood supply along with coverage that is bulkier and more reliable than that obtained by a split-thickness graft, particularly in an irradiated field.

The elliptical resections are oriented vertically or horizontally, preferably the latter, depending on the location of the primary tumor.

After skin incision, flaps are raised as in the modified radical mastectomy. Dissection is carried superiorly to the clavicle, laterally to the anterior border of the latissimus dorsi, medially to the lateral sternal border, and inferiorly to 3 cm below the

101

inframammary fold. The deltopectoral groove is then located superiorly by identifying the cephalic vein. This plane of cleavage is opened widely and the tendinous insertion of the pectoralis major into the humerus is identified and divided with the electrocautery (Fig. 8-1*A*). The clavipectoral fascia is opened, thus exposing the pectoralis minor, whose attachment to the coracoid process is severed (Fig. 8-1*B*). Both pectoral muscles are retracted inferiorly, thus exposing the axilla. The loose fat overlying the brachial plexus is swept inferiorly and the axillary vein is exposed. The fascia overlying the vein is incised and all tributaries are ligated. The axillary tissue is then carefully dissected inferiorly, exposing and preserving the long thoracic nerve as it passes medially over the serratus anterior. The thoracodorsal nerve is also iden-

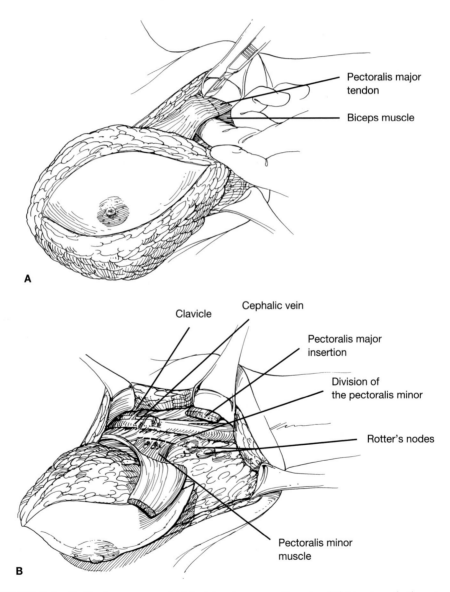

**FIGURE 8-1.** Radical mastectomy. (**A**) Incising the pectoralis major. (**B**) Ligation of tributaries of the axillary vein.

tified and protected laterally, and the axillary fat pad between the two nerves is dissected free of the subscapularis muscle.

The breast and both pectoral muscles are then dissected medially. As the perforating branches of the internal mammary artery are identified, they are doubly ligated. The attachments of the pectoralis major to the ribs are severed with the electrocautery and the dissection is carried inferiorly to the rectus fascia. The breast is removed and sent without fixation to pathology. Suction drains (Jackson-Pratt) are employed as in a modified radical mastectomy, and the wound is closed in the same fashion. If necessary, a split-thickness skin graft or an alternative reconstruction is performed to cover the resultant chest wall defects. A pressure dressing is applied to minimize adverse motion of a skin graft.

# *Part* IV
## Postmastectomy Reconstruction

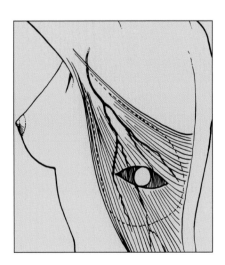

*Atlas of Techniques in Breast Surgery,*
by William Silen, W. Earle Matory, Jr. and Susan M. Love.
Lippincott-Raven Publishers, Philadelphia, © 1996.

# Chapter

# 9

# Questions, Controversies, and Decisions

S everal issues concerning reconstruction confront the patient, the general and plastic surgeons, and the oncologist, the most important of which are discussed in the following text.

## ✦ WHY UNDERGO BREAST RECONSTRUCTION?

All patients undergoing partial or total ablation of the breast for benign or malignant disease are potential candidates for breast reconstruction. In the past, patients with relatively poor prognosis were not considered to be suitable for breast reconstruction but both quality of life and chances of survival are key factors in making a decision to carry out reconstruction.

The devastating emotional impact of mastectomy is lessened considerably by early or delayed reconstruction. The earlier the reconstruction, the less severe the depression that follows the ablative surgery.[1-3] Thus, any patient anticipating or incurring deformity to the breast is a candidate for immediate or delayed breast reconstruction.

## ✦ PATIENT AND SOCIETAL RESPONSE TO BREAST RECONSTRUCTION

A study by McCraw and coworkers[4] analyzed patient satisfaction with results after breast reconstruction with tissue expanders or transverse rectus abdominis myocutaneous (TRAM) flaps. More than 98% of patients were satisfied with the outcome after TRAM and 85% were pleased after tissue expansion followed by

107

implant placement. Some of the causes of dissatisfaction of patients after breast reconstruction are shown in Table 9-1. This experience mirrors that of other surgeons throughout the United States. Aesthetic outcome continues to improve as plastic surgeons and general surgeons refine ablative and reconstructive techniques.

More than 90% of postreconstruction patients noted improvement or no deterioration in walking, swimming, aerobics, jogging, tennis, or skiing after rectus muscle transfer.[5] Ninety-three percent considered the rectus flap reconstruction to be worthwhile and more than 96% would recommend the procedure to others.

Functional recovery continues to become more rapid and more complete, commensurate with improved technologic refinement by oncologic and reconstructive surgeons. Table 9-2 outlines the anticipated hospital course and recovery patterns after various reconstructive alternatives.

## ✦ WHO SHOULD NOT UNDERGO BREAST RECONSTRUCTION?

The only absolute contraindication to breast reconstruction is medical illness that may compromise patient safety during and immediately after the reconstruction. Although physiologic age influences the medical risks of reconstruction, the aging citizenry of the United States is far more vigorous and motivated toward postmastectomy reconstruction than patients in the past. We have performed reconstruction on patients as old as 96. In contrast, there are some 60-year-old individuals who would not tolerate a brief anesthetic, much less a 1- to 6-hour extension for breast reconstruction.

The extent of local or systemic malignant disease is not a contraindication to reconstruction unless there is some physiologic compromise that will adversely affect anesthetic safety. The heavy smoker should eliminate all nicotine exposure at least 2 weeks before transfer of a myocutaneous flap or implant reconstruction. The obese

**TABLE 9-1**

Causes of Patient Dissatisfaction With Breast Reconstruction

| Cause of Dissatisfaction | Tissue Expander and Implant (n = 55) | Transverse Rectus Abdominis Musculocutaneous Flap (n = 74) |
|---|---|---|
| Pain | 6 | 11 |
| Asymmetry | 28 | 6 |
| Shape and contour | 22 | 4 |
| Prolonged reconstruction | 17 | 8 |
| Expander discomfort | 8 | 0 |
| Abdominal contour | 0 | 15 |

Reprinted with permission from McCraw JB et al: An early appraisal of the methods of tissue expansion and the transverse rectus abdominis musculocutaneous flap in reconstruction of the breast following mastectomy. Ann Plast Surg 1987;18:93.

**TABLE 9-2**

Reconstructive Options After Mastectomy

| Operative Time (h) | Hospital Stay (d) | Postoperative Visits | Return to Work (wks) | Indications and Patient Presentation | Contraindications |
|---|---|---|---|---|---|
| **Submuscular implants** | | | | | |
| 1 | 2–3 | 4 | 1–3 | Small-breasted | Not used after large skin resection |
| **Tissue expander** | | | | | |
| 1 | 2–3 | 8 | 1–3 | Small- or medium-breasted | — |
| **Latissimus dorsi (muscle implant)** | | | | | |
| 3 | 3–5 | 4 | 2–4 | Small and medium-breasts | Not advised in avid swimmers or golfers |
| **Transverse rectus abdominis myocutaneous flaps** | | | | | |
| 5 | 5–7 | 4 | 2–4 | Small, medium, and large breasts | Avoid in patients with severe or chronic back pain |
| **Free tissue transfer** | | | | | |
| 5–7 | 5–10 | 4 | 2–4 | Small, medium, and large breasts | — |

patient may benefit from weight reduction. Although operative techniques can be varied to optimize vascularity of the skin or myocutaneous flaps, the choice of reconstructive alternatives in the smoker and in the obese patient is sharply restricted. Seromas, hematomas, and infection are more likely in these patients, both at the site of chest wall reconstruction and at the donor site.

## ✦ WILL RECONSTRUCTION MASK LOCAL SKIN, SUBCUTANEOUS, OR CHEST WALL RECURRENCE?

Most local–regional recurrences of breast cancer develop within the native skin and subcutaneous tissues adjacent to the mastectomy and flap reconstruction sites.[6,7] Slavin and coworkers[7] reviewed a series of recurrences among 161 patients undergoing myocutaneous flap reconstructions after mastectomy (Table 9-3). With a mean follow-up of 5.4 years, 17 (10.6%) local recurrences were noted—14 of 120 (11.7%) after primary mastectomy with reconstruction and three of 41 (7.3%) after salvage mastectomy. The propensity for recurrence increased as the stage of the primary cancer increased (see Table 9-3). The diagnosis of local recurrence was not delayed nor was there a compromise of patient survival as a result of implant or myocutaneous flap reconstruction. Recurrences are treated with chemotherapy, local radiation, or excision of the lesion. Removal of the breast reconstruction is rarely indicated.

**TABLE 9-3**

Local Recurrence According to Stage

| | Patients (n) | Patients With Local Recurrence | |
|---|---|---|---|
| | | (n) | (%) |
| 0–I | 98 | 0 | 0 |
| II | 43 | 6 | 14 |
| III | 19 | 10 | 52.6 |
| IV | 1 | 1 | 100 |
| **TOTAL** | **161** | **17** | |

Reprinted with permission from Slavin S, Love S, Goldwyn R. Recurrent breast cancer following immediate reconstruction with myocutaneous flaps. Plast Reconstr Surg 1994;93:1191.

## ✦ TIMING OF RECONSTRUCTION

The devastating emotional impact of mastectomy may be lessened by early reconstruction and the earlier the reconstruction, the less severe the depression that follows ablative surgery.[1] From a technical standpoint, overall outcome is improved with reconstruction at the time of mastectomy: skin flaps are softer and free of chronic fibrosis, inframammary fold is visible and easier to recreate, and nearly exact dimensions of the tissue that has been removed with a mastectomy can be replaced. Many authorities are strong advocates of the effectiveness and safety of immediate breast reconstruction.[8-12] Immediate reconstruction offers several advantages: (1) the psychological impact of breast loss is reduced, (2) the cost of postmastectomy reconstruction is lessened, (3) the dimensions of the mastectomy specimen can be precisely assessed and replaced, thus creating a contour similar to that before mastectomy.

If for some reason immediate reconstruction is not performed, delayed breast restoration can be performed after healing is complete and the acute reaction of the mastectomy has resolved. Rarely is delayed reconstruction possible before 3 months after surgery. The chest wall must be soft, pliable, nontender, and without evidence of infection. When any of these factors are present, aesthetic outcome and the chances for an uncomplicated recovery are compromised.

## ✦ PLASTIC SURGERY CONSULTATION

It is crucial that the reconstructive surgeon be consulted as early as possible before surgery. Evaluation of the patient for suitability and reconstructive alternatives requires explanation, time for planning, and time for insurance approval. Note that implants may be on back-order from the manufacturers, and custom implants may require 4 to 6 weeks for delivery.

## ✦ WILL POSTMASTECTOMY RADIATION OR CHEMOTHERAPY BE COMPROMISED OR DELAYED?

Regardless of the method chosen, reconstructive considerations must not hinder the treatment of the breast cancer. Prosthetic or myocutaneous flap reconstruction does not interfere with chemotherapy or radiation therapy. Implants do not block or enhance the absorption of radiation.[7] There is no evidence that the silicone prosthesis impairs the systemic immunologic response.[13]

Wound complications that may be encountered after mastectomy rarely delay postmastectomy therapy. Partial flap necrosis or infection is usually resolved within a 1- to 2-week period. Patients with a resultant open wound can undergo chemotherapy as long as bacterial contamination has been minimized and any closed contaminated space is adequately drained.

## ✦ THE OPPOSITE BREAST

Procedures designed to allow the uninvolved breast to match the reconstructed one are useful under certain circumstances. The patient must be given the opportunity to review surgical options. Any surgical manipulation of the opposite breast can potentially cause changes in sensation and distortions or calcifications that could compromise future diagnostic efforts. Such calcifications induced by a surgical procedure are generally benign and are usually larger than those noted in cancerous lesions. Breast reductions, mastopexies, and augmentations in the opposite breast have been performed consistently for the last 10 years, without substantive evidence that subsequent diagnostic efforts are compromised although controlled trials have not been done to examine this question.

## ✦ MAMMOGRAPHY AND BREAST IMPLANTS

Several studies have implied that breast implantation may impair the pre- or postmastectomy mammogram by 20% to 40%. Visualization is optimized by distracting the breast away from the implant and simultaneously pushing the implant posteriorly (Fig. 9-1). Distraction techniques have limited benefit in the small-breasted nonptotic patient (less than 300 g) or after the development of severe distortion due to capsular contraction.

Early work by Matory and coworkers[14] suggests that visualization can be improved by deflating implants before mammography (Fig. 9-2), with reinflation immediately after. Numerous other options are being analyzed in an effort to optimize mammographic accuracy in this population.

## ✦ SHOULD ONE BE CONCERNED ABOUT A PROSTHETIC RECONSTRUCTION?

Considerable controversy and media attention regarding breast-implant devices have surfaced during the past 5 years.[13,15,16] Prosthetic devices continue to be a mainstay in medical care, particularly for breast reconstruction. Such devices serve as substitutes for human de-

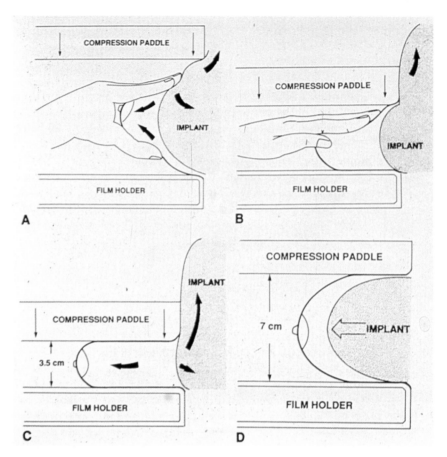

**FIGURE 9-1.** Radiologic visualization is optimized by distracting the breast away from the implant and simultaneously pushing the implant posteriorly. (Matory WE Jr, D'Orsi C, Moss L. Improved mammographic imaging using tissue expanders for breast augmentation. Ann Plast Surg 1994; 33(2):119.)

ficiencies or deformations but are not without fault. There are defined risks of implantation, including infection (1%), bleeding (1%), implant leakage or deflation (2% to 35%), silicone migration (less than 1%), capsular contracture (15% to 35%), calcium deposits (3% to 5%), loss of nipple or breast sensation (1%), and interference with mammography (20%). Untoward events accompanying breast prostheses are far less frequent and less severe than those associated with prosthetic heart valves or penile implants, however.

In addition, unknown lifelong risks may be present but are as yet undetected. These devices have been used for only 30 years. It has been suggested that connective-tissue disorders, cancer, and birth defects may be related to implants but these associations have not been proved conclusively. Two newer studies demonstrate divergent data related to the problem of connective-tissue disorders. Gabriel and coworkers,[17] in a large retrospective population-based study, found no association between connective-tissue disorders and breast implants. Conversely, Smalley and coworkers have found that silicone seems to induce an immune response but whether this response has any clinical significance is unclear. The Scleroderma Task Force of the American Medical Association has determined that there is no epidemiologic correlation between silicone implants and autoimmune disease. The overall record of more than 4 million women

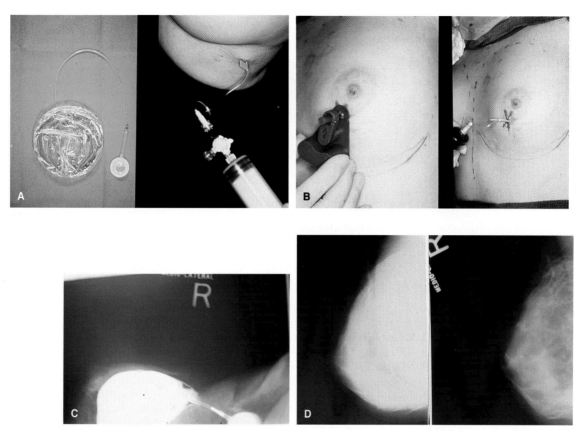

**FIGURE 9-2.**   (**A** and **B**) Tissue expander valves are entered with a fine gauge needle. Valves are identified by palpation or with the use of a magnet. (**C**) A remote valve expander is illustrated with valve positioning in the axilla. (**D**) A significant radiopacity in a breast with a saline expander. Following deflation, breast parenchyma is more easily evaluated.

undergoing breast implant procedures has been exceptionally good but patients and healthcare workers should be made aware of several concerns, which are outlined in the section entitled Breast Reconstruction, Prosthetic Devices (see Chapter 10). Many other issues have been raised regarding silicone and saline implants. The possibility of an association between silicone implants and an increased risk of autoimmune disease has prompted the Food and Drug Administration (FDA) to look into the safety of the breast prosthesis.[15] In January 1992, on the basis of uncertainty and worries, the FDA temporarily banned the use of gel-filled implants until sufficient documentation exists of their safety and effectiveness. In April 1992, the FDA ruled that breast implants with silicone gel would be made available only through a controlled clinical trial in patients undergoing breast reconstruction or in those having prior saline or silicone gel implants. Many authorities have criticized the lack of a scientific basis for these FDA decisions.[13,16] Breast-implant controversies have drawn attention to the need for more knowledge and experience to develop safe and effective compatible materials (Table 9-4).

Ongoing research by immunologists, basic scientists, and plastic surgeons is directed toward enhancement of the safety of silicone and saline implant devices. Any patient contemplating a breast implantation must weigh the advantages of improved self-esteem and self-image with the potential trade-offs (i.e., the inherent risks of

**TABLE 9-4**

Ideal Implant

| | |
|---|---|
| Impervious to tissue fluid | Nonallergic |
| Chemically inert | Resistant to mechanical strains |
| Nonirritating | Capable of fabrication as desired |
| Noncarcinogenic | Sterilizable |

prosthetic devices). Although individual risks are relatively infrequent, one must anticipate that in a normal lifespan, some additional procedure may become necessary to address one or more of the listed untoward events.

## REFERENCES

1. Schain WS, Jacobs E, Wellisch DK. Psychosocial issues in breast reconstruction: intrapsychic, interpersonal, and practical concerns. Clin Plast Surg 1984;11:237.
2. Goldwyn RM. Breast reconstruction after mastectomy. N Engl J Med 1987;317:1711.
3. Radovan C. Breast reconstruction after mastectomy using a temporary expander. Plast Reconstr Surg 1982;69:195.
4. McCraw JB, Horton CE, Grossman JA, et al. An early appraisal of the methods of tissue expansion and the transverse rectus abdomins musculocutaneous flap in reconstruction of the breast following mastectomy. Ann Plast Surg 1987;18:93.
5. Mizgala C, Hartrampf CR Jr, Bennett K. Assessment of abdominal wall surgery after pedicled TRAM flap surgery: 5 to 7 year follow-up of 150 consecutive patients. Plast Recontr Surg 1994;93:988.
6. Johnson CH, van Heerden JA, Donohue JH, et al. Oncological aspects of immediate breast reconstruction following mastectomy for malignancy. Arch Surg 1989;124:819.
7. Slavin S, Love S, Goldwyn R. Recurrent breast cancer following immediate reconstruction with myocutaneous flaps. Plast Reconstr Surg 1994;93:1191.
8. Georgiade GS. Immediate reconstruction of the breast following modified radical mastectomy for carcinoma of the breast. Clin Plast Surg 1984;11:383.
9. Frazier TG, Noone RB. An objective analysis of immediate simultaneous reconstruction in the treatment of primary carcinoma of the breast. Cancer 1985;55:1202.
10. Georgiade GS, Riefkhol R, Cox E, et al. Long-term clinical outcome of immediate reconstruction after mastectomy. Plast Reconstr Surg 1985;76:415.
11. Webster DJT, Mansel RE, Hughes IE. Immediate reconstruction of the breast after mastectomy: is it safe? Cancer 1984;53:1416.
12. Noone RB, Murphy JB, Spear SL, et al. A 6-year experience with immediate reconstruction after mastectomy for cancer. Plast Reconstr Surg 1985;76:258.
13. Fisher JC. The silicone controversy—when will science prevail? N Engl J Med 1992;326:1696.
14. Matory WE Jr, D'Orsi C, Moss L. Improving mammographic imaging by using tissue expanders for augmentation mammoplasty. Ann Plast Surg 1994;33:1.
15. Kessler DA. The basis of FDA's decision on breast implants. N Engl J Med 1992;326:1713.
16. Angell M. Breast implants—protection or paternalism? N Engl J Med 1992;326:1695.
17. Gabriel SE, O'Fallon WM, Kurland LT, et al. Risk of connective-tissue diseases and other disorders after breast implantation. N Engl J Med 1994;33:1697.

114

*Atlas of Techniques in Breast Surgery,*
by William Silen, W. Earle Matory, Jr. and Susan M. Love.
Lippincott-Raven Publishers, Philadelphia, © 1996.

# *Chapter* 10

# Types of Breast Reconstruction

T he following techniques are used for immediate or delayed reconstruction of the breast:

Placement of prosthetic devices
    Submuscular implant
    Submuscular tissue expander
Autologous reconstruction
    Latissimus dorsi myocutaneous flap with or without a submuscular implant
    Rectus abdominis myocutaneous (RAM) flap
    Free-tissue transfer (free flap)

## ✦ *PROSTHETIC DEVICES*

### *Placement of a Submuscular Implant*

Snyderman and Guthrie[1] in 1971 reported the first case of postmastectomy reconstruction by subcutaneous placement of a silicone implant under the chest wall skin. In the early days, the limited size of the skin envelope, the marginal circulation of the remaining breast skin, or both often prevented proper implant volume and positioning to match the opposite breast, and capsular contracture was common.

As reconstructions became more widespread in the 70s, technical improvements clearly enhanced the results of these procedures (Fig. 10-1*A* and *B*). The incidence of capsular contracture decreased dramatically when implants were placed under the chest wall musculature, providing an improved local blood supply.[2]

115

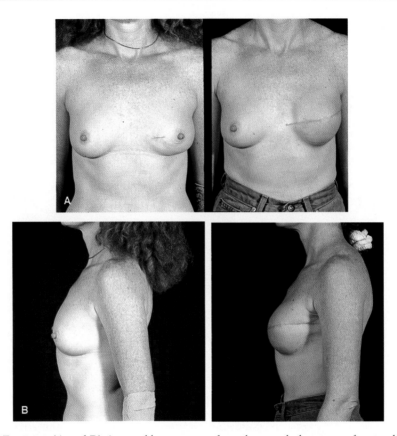

**FIGURE 10-1.** (**A** and **B**) Acceptable outcomes after subpectoral placement of an implant after mastectomy.

## INDICATIONS

Submuscular implants are appropriate in instances wherein a minimal amount of skin has been resected at the mastectomy or in individuals with very small breasts needing only a modicum of breast fullness. Patients who have excess skin (i.e., ptosis) also benefit from implantation, with or without contralateral matching reduction or mastopexy. Adequate skin and muscle to cover the implant without tension of the wound closure is a requisite for success. One must ensure adequate coverage of the implant to diminish the likelihood of implant exposure and extrusion. Late postoperative pericapsular fibrosis is more likely after delayed than after immediate reconstruction with a nonexpander implant. Smooth silicone-enveloped prostheses tend to promote periprosthetic capsular contracture. Periprosthetic fibrosis is theoretically minimized by making the surface of these devices rough or irregular. Thus, use of polyurethane-covered and textured silicone prosthetics has resulted in a diminished incidence of capsular contracture.[3] Polyurethane devices have been removed from the market, however, because of concerns about breakdown products of the polyurethane. Use of other types of textured implants continues to increase in popularity and appears to effectively diminish capsular contracture rates.

## POSITIONING AND PREPARATION

With the patient in the supine position, sterile preparation should be from posterior axillary line to posterior axillary line and from clavicle to mid-epigastrium. The contralateral breast must be prepared within the same field, so that symmetry can be assessed easily. A plastic adherent drape or towel may be used to cover the contralateral breast during the mastectomy. The arms are abducted to 90 degrees symmetrically and secured to the arm boards with gauze roll or biased stockinet. The axilla is prepared within the field. Perioperative antibiotics are appropriate when implants are used because bacterial contamination may lead to infection or significant capsular contracture. The pectoralis major and minor and the serratus muscles must be carefully preserved, so that these can be used for coverage of the implant.

## OPERATIVE PROCEDURE

After mastectomy, the bundles of the pectoralis major are separated along the direction of the fibers for a distance long enough to insert the prosthesis. Using a lighted retractor, a submuscular plane is dissected bluntly to the second intercostal space superiorly. The anterior serratus and the rectus muscle may be sharply dissected from the ribs inferiorly to 2 cm below the inframammary fold. The medial inferior fibers of the pectoralis major are released from the sternal insertion to allow medial positioning of the implant. Total muscle coverage of the implant is not always possible but is nevertheless desirable. Incomplete muscle coverage beneath the mastectomy incision may suffice if skin flaps are of adequate thickness. Sizers are used to determine the optimal implant size. Interrupted 3-0 absorbable sutures are placed in the separated fibers of the pectoralis major but not yet tied. Before implant placement, drains are placed in the lateral inferior pocket and brought out through stab incisions in the axilla or flank. The implant is then placed in the submuscular pocket (Fig. 10-2*A* and *B*) after hemostasis has been confirmed, and the sutures are tied. The skin is approximated using interrupted 3-0 absorbable sutures and a running cutaneous 5-0 polypropylene suture. Vaseline-impregnated gauze is applied to the skin incision along with an overlying dry, sterile dressing.

Drains are usually removed within 5 days to diminish bacterial contamination of the implant. A compression dressing may be helpful in diminishing the likelihood of hematoma or seroma. A custom-fitted brassiere can be ordered preoperatively to provide support. When the latter is unavailable, an Ace bandage wrapped circumferentially about the chest serves the same purpose. Ice compression garments are often used to diminish postoperative swelling, discomfort, and bleeding.

## COMPLICATIONS

The most common risk of immediate reconstruction of the breast with a submuscular implant is severe capsular contracture about the prosthesis. The incidence of this complication has gradually decreased from 40% to 60% in the early days of the procedure to 2% to 11%.[4,5] Periprosthetic contracture may lead to discomfort, displacement, and resultant asymmetry. The trauma of the surgical dissection, pericapsular hematoma, and bacterial contamination have been proposed as contributing factors to capsular formation. When these symptoms occur, an additional operation may be required to release the capsule or reposition the implant (Fig. 10-3).

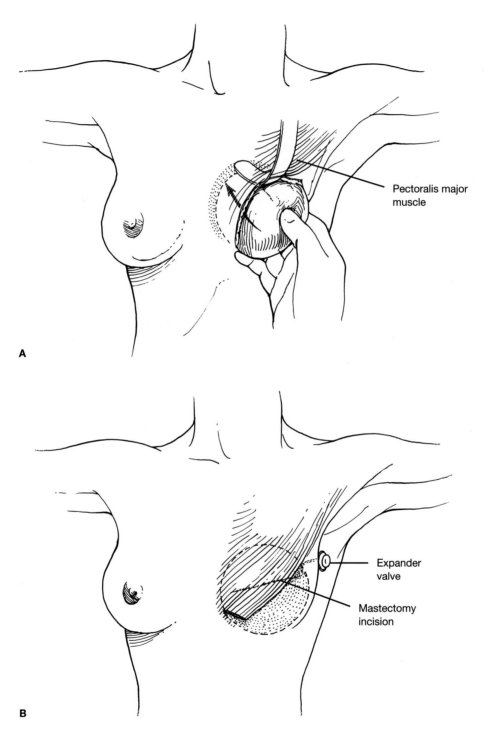

A

B

**FIGURE 10-2.** Placing an implant.

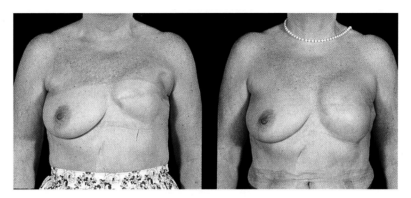

**FIGURE 10-3.** Marked improvement of appearance after releasing and excising the scar of a capsular implant followed by repositioning of the implant.

Hematoma, infection, and pneumothorax after the submuscular dissection are relatively infrequent, occurring in fewer than 5%. Implant extrusion due to infection or inadequate muscle coverage may require removal of the implant to effect resolution of the infection. Subsequent replacement of an implant or use of alternate forms of reconstruction may then be necessary. Implant deflation or leakage may occur with saline and gel implants in 1% to 10% and in 1% of patients, respectively. These latter problems require implant replacement. The added operative time of about 1 hour for the use of an implant does not add any clinically significant anesthetic risk to that of mastectomy (see Table 9-2 in Chap. 9).

## Placement of a Submuscular Tissue Expander

Radovan[6] in 1982 published a series of 68 subcutaneous expander devices that were used to stretch the remaining skin after mastectomy. Several authors have subsequently reported successful use of tissue expanders, which has become one of the most commonly used forms of reconstruction.[6–10]

### INDICATIONS

Tissue expansion is most useful in patients having an A-, B-, or C-size bra who have adequate skin to close the chest wall defect and who lack contralateral ptosis. When contralateral ptosis or a large contralateral breast is present, a simultaneous mastopexy or breast reduction should be considered to help match each side. Breast contouring can be closer to that of the contralateral breast when a conservative skin resection is performed at the time of mastectomy. Serial inflation of the tissue expander stretches the residual amount of skin to optimize symmetry.

### SURGICAL PROCEDURE AND FOLLOW-UP

As described for submuscular placement of an implant, preparation of both breasts is indicated. A submuscular dissection is performed in a manner similar to that for the submuscular breast implant. The feeding valve of the device may be located on the implant itself or as a separate or remote valve. A small pocket is dissected laterally to hide the remote valve in the axilla. Saline is instilled into the expander after positioning of the implant and muscle closure while observing to make certain that there is no undue tension on the skin. Drains and compression dressings are used in a manner similar to that described for submuscular implant placement.

Further implant expansion begins 2 weeks later with weekly instillation of 100 to 200 mL saline, adjusted to avoid patient discomfort. The volume is gradually increased to 50% to 100% more than the desired final implant volume (Fig. 10-4*A*). Overexpansion ensures adequate long-term skin volume (Fig. 10-4*B*). The additional volume is maintained for as long as the patient is able to tolerate it to maximize maturation of the periprosthetic capsule that occurs around all prostheses (up to 6 months but usually 2 months). The tissue expander is then deflated to the de-

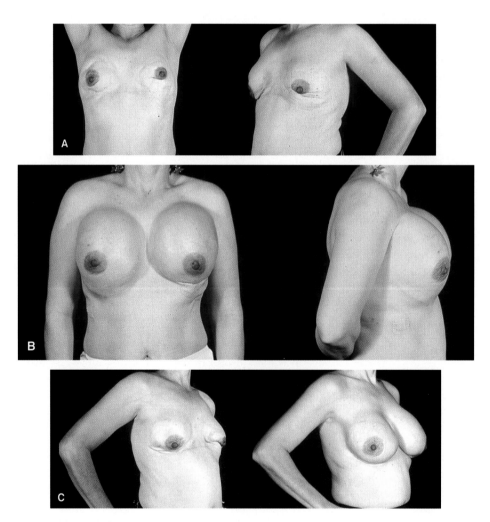

**FIGURE 10-4.** (**A**) Appearance after bilateral subcutaneous mastectomy. (**B**) After insertion of bilateral tissue expanders under the pectoralis muscle and the rectus fascia. Inflation to 1500 mL in each breast was maintained for 6 months. (**C**) After placement of permanent implants.

sired size. It can be replaced by a standard implant with the desired volume at the time of nipple reconstruction. Expansion normally takes 4 to 6 weeks, with subsequent deflation to the desired volume at about 3 to 4 months postmastectomy (Fig. 10-4*C*). Expansion can be performed during a course of radiation or chemotherapy, if necessary.

### COMPLICATIONS

The most common complication after mastectomy and tissue expansion is that of periprosthetic capsular contracture, with an incidence of 5.8% to 13%.[2,11,12] With the use of less extensive ablative techniques (e.g., skin-sparing mastectomies), the incidence of capsular contracture, implant infection, and exposure has been decreasing.

Capsular contracture is less likely after tissue expansion than after placement of a fixed-size nonexpandable implant.[2,4,11] Release of a contracture may be indicated in 5% to 15% of these postmastectomy reconstructions and is usually performed at the time of nipple reconstruction. Deflation of the implant may occur during needle placement for each of the weekly expansions. The likelihood of this risk is small with the remote valve or with the magnet-guided on-site valve. Malposition of the expander valve is an infrequent occurrence that can be addressed easily in an office procedure. Other potential complications of the use of expanders are similar in kind and incidence to those of the standard fixed implant. Discomfort of the patient during expansion can be considerable.

## ✦ AUTOLOGOUS RECONSTRUCTION

Immediate reconstruction with myocutaneous flaps enables precise replacement of the amount of skin excised at the time of total mastectomy. Myocutaneous flaps provide well-vascularized tissue to replace the breast mound or to cover an underlying implant. Patients who have had a sizable skin resection, a radical mastectomy, or damage to the lateral or medial pectoral nerves usually require transposition of skin and muscle to replace the atrophic or surgically absent pectoralis major muscle or overlying skin.

### Latissimus Dorsi Myocutaneous Flap Reconstruction With or Without Submuscular Implant

#### INDICATIONS

The latissimus dorsi is a large fan-shaped muscle, extending from the spinous processes of the seventh through the twelfth thoracic vertebrae, the thoracolumbar fascia, and the posterior third of the iliac crest to a tendinous insertion into the lateral humerus. The muscle adducts the humerus and rotates the shoulder posteriorly. Alternative motor units of the shoulder perform similar functions, making the latissimus an expendable muscle unit. In active golfers and swimmers, the functional deficit of loss of the latissimus muscle may impair these activities to some extent.

### POSITIONING AND PREPARATION

While awake, the patient is placed in the sitting position, so that the incisions can be outlined to reside within the bra line (Fig. 10-5*A* and *B*).

The lateral decubitus position allows mastectomy and muscle flap harvest within the same field (Fig. 10-6). A bean bag for the trunk in addition to pillows to support the knees are used to stabilize the patient. The trunk and extremities are carefully padded. The ipsilateral arm is prepared within the field to allow posterior rotation of the shoulder for mastectomy and axillary dissection and allow anterior rotation for latissimus harvest. The sterile preparation should extend from the mid-back to the midline anteriorly.

### OPERATIVE TECHNIQUE

On completion of the mastectomy and harvest of the muscle flap, the patient is repositioned into the supine position to allow visualization of the contralateral breast for comparison and optimization.

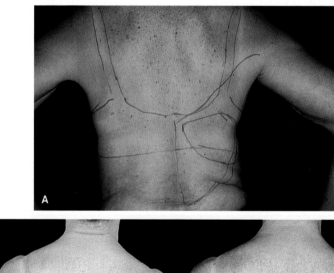

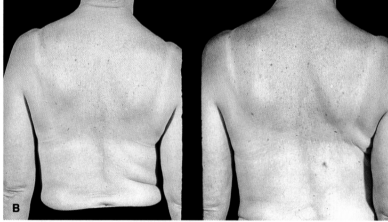

**FIGURE 10-5.** (**A**) In the sitting position, skin incisions are outlined so that scars will be hidden within the bra line. (**B**) The donor defect is illustrated.

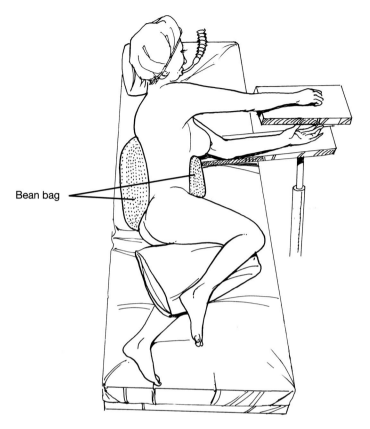

**FIGURE 10-6.**  Positioning for immediate reconstruction using a latissimus flap.

The thoracodorsal neurovascular bundle supplies the latissimus dorsi muscle, and musculocutaneous perforators supply the overlying skin. If a skin-sparing mastectomy has been performed, a small skin island is used (Fig. 10-7*A* and *B*). Skin flaps up to 8 to 10 cm in width can be employed without yielding a widened or disfiguring scar on the back (see Fig. 10-5*A* and *B*). The skin island and accompanying muscle are rotated to the anterior chest, based on the thoracodorsal blood supply.

In the small-breasted patient, a large skin island on the latissimus dorsi can be harvested for autologous reconstruction of the breast by extending the skin island superiorly, anterolaterally, and inferiorly (Fig. 10-8). The resultant fleur-de-lis pattern allows primary closure of the donor defect, although the scar may be more visible than with a smaller flap of this kind, especially when an inferior extension of the incision below the bra line has been used. The skin resection of the total mastectomy is outlined by the general surgeon. A template duplicating the exact amount of skin to be excised is made to document the dimensions and orientation of the defect. The latissimus flap can be raised during the completion of the total mastectomy. Using the template, the skin overlying the latissimus muscle is outlined with a marking pen. Preoperatively, the position of the bra has been determined, and an effort is made to position the scar underneath the bra strap. The skin island,

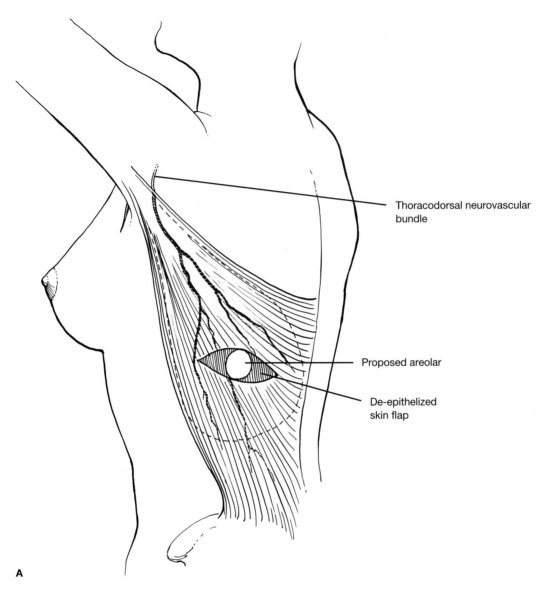

Thoracodorsal neurovascular bundle

Proposed areolar

De-epithelized skin flap

**A**

**FIGURE 10-7.** (A) Small skin island on a latissimus dorsi muscle flap. (B) Latissimus flap transposed to the underlying chest, with an underlying tissue expander.

along with the underlying latissimus dorsi muscle, is dissected free as follows. The lateral border of the latissimus is identified, and the muscle is mobilized by dissecting deep to it and transecting the thoracolumbar fascia and medial origin of the muscle. The mobilization of the muscle is carried cephalad to where the thoracodorsal vessels are identified, about 10 to 12 cm from the axillary vein. Care must be taken to preserve the communication of the thoracodorsal vessels with the serratus anterior collateral vessel, especially when the thoracodorsal pedicle has been transected during the mastectomy. Sutures between the dermis of the skin island and the muscle are placed to prevent avulsion of the skin from the latissimus. A sub-

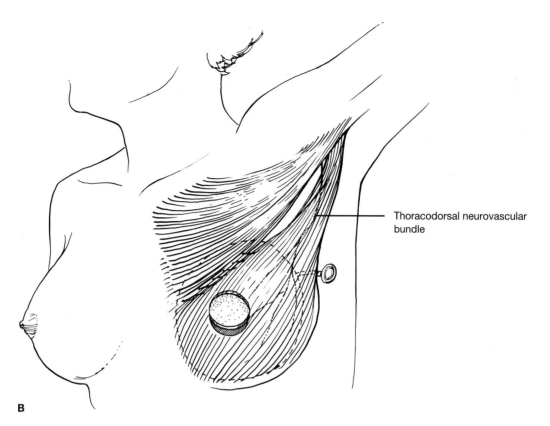

Thoracodorsal neurovascular
bundle

**B**

**FIGURE 10-7.** *(Continued)*

cutaneous pocket is made high in the axilla to allow anterior transposition of the myocutaneous flap. The humeral insertion of the latissimus dorsi can be divided if needed to facilitate transposition of the flap. The insertion can also be repositioned to recreate an anterior axillary fold if the pectoralis muscle has been removed during a radical mastectomy.

Hemostasis is confirmed, closed suction catheters are placed, and the posterior skin incision is closed with interrupted 3-0 and 4-0 absorbable sutures in the dermis, followed by a running cutaneous polypropylene suture. A dry, sterile dressing is applied to the back, and the patient is rotated to the supine position.

A pocket deep to the pectoralis major is dissected to accommodate a synthetic implant, if such is to be used. Ideally, the latissimus skin island is placed as far inferiorly as possible to reproduce contralateral ptosis and to minimize visibility of the scar. The latissimus is sutured inferiorly to the lower border of the pectoralis and to the rectus fascia along the inframammary crease. Superiorly, the latissimus may be sutured to the fascia along the clavicle and to the lateral border of the pectoralis major. When an implant is to be inserted, sizers are used to match the volume of the contralateral breast, and a suitable implant is placed in the subpectoral pocket. Contralateral breast reduction, enlargement, or mastopexy can also be performed at the same time if the patient desires. The skin is closed temporarily with sutures or staples. The head of the operating table is raised to assess symmetry;

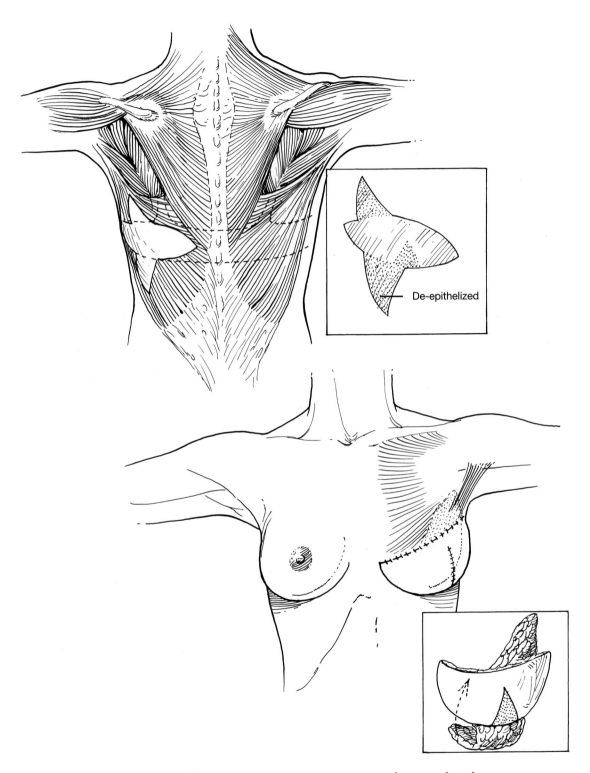

De-epithelized

**FIGURE 10-8.** A fully autologous breast reconstruction using a myocutaneous latissimus dorsi skin island transposed to the anterior chest without an underlying implant.

once this has been achieved, the dermis and skin are approximated. Before skin closure, drains are positioned to evacuate the donor site, axilla, and the submuscular or supramuscular pockets or both. Arm exercises are usually delayed for 72 to 96 hours after surgery to diminish seroma formation and vasospasm in the thoracodorsal vessels.

### COMPLICATIONS

The latissimus dorsi myocutaneous flap is sturdy and has an excellent blood supply. Skin or muscle loss is infrequent, even in the smoker or obese patient. Capsular contracture and other complications associated with an implant occur with the same frequency as after simple placement of an implant. Seroma formation at the latissimus dorsi donor site may develop in 30% to 50% of the cases. Serial aspiration minimizes the formation of a pseudobursa. The donor defect is usually well hidden, thin-lined, and beneath the bra or bathing suit, although occasionally the scar widens and may become visible.

## Rectus Abdominis Myocutaneous Flap Reconstruction

### INDICATIONS

The rectus myocutaneous flap also allows replacement of skin and breast mass. The construction of this flap is a lengthier and more complex procedure but it has distinct advantages:

1. The rectus allows transfer of adequate bulk to replace the missing breast without use of an implant in most patients.
2. In patients with a large contralateral breast, the missing breast mass and the natural ptosis can often be duplicated.
3. The abdominal wall is recontoured simultaneously (Fig. 10-9*A* and *B*).

The use of autogenous tissue yields a softer and more natural-appearing reconstruction. By duplicating the amount of skin and parenchyma removed in the mastectomy, excellent symmetry can be achieved. As much as 2 to 4 units of blood may be lost during the combined procedure and hence, transfusion of previously banked autologous blood should be considered. The transverse rectus abdominis myocutaneous flap (TRAM) is contraindicated in heavy smokers, morbidly obese patients, or in patients having compromised cutaneous circulation. Cessation of smoking 2 weeks before surgery and throughout the postoperative course decreases the likelihood of postoperative fat necrosis. Because the cutaneous island in the morbidly obese patient appears to have impaired circulation, the vertical rectus abdominis myocutaneous flap (VRAM) may be more suitable for these patients.

Because the rectus muscle stabilizes the back, TRAM or VRAM flaps may be contraindicated in the patient who has chronic back pain. A prior Kocher's incision that has resulted in ligation of the right superior epigastric vessels eliminates the possibility of using an ipsilateral RAM, in which case the contralateral RAM or an inferiorly based free flap can be employed.

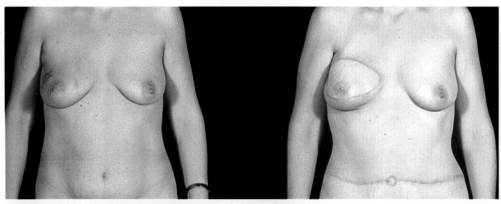

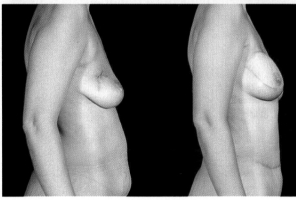

**FIGURE 10-9.** Good breast reconstruction concomitant with abdominal flattening can be achieved with the unilateral pedicled transverse rectus abdominus myocutaneous flap.

### PREPARATION AND POSITIONING

The patient is placed in the supine position, with the gatch of the operation table at the hips. This allows flexion of the hips to minimize tension at the time of the abdominal closure.

The sterile preparation extends from the clavicle to the mid-pubis and bilaterally to the posterior axillary line, including both breasts. A sterile drape or towel is applied to the contralateral breast.

### OPERATIVE PROCEDURE

Total mastectomy is completed. The wound is irrigated and hemostasis is confirmed. A template of the resected mastectomy skin is placed to outline a transverse or longitudinal ellipse of skin on the abdomen overlying the rectus muscle. Skin may be harvested from just above, at, or just below the umbilicus. Most myocutaneous perforating vessels are located in close proximity to the umbilicus, making this area the most reliable source of abdominal skin (Fig. 10-10A). The skin flap is elevated, taking care to preserve its attachments to the rectus fascia and muscle. The rectus muscle is transected inferior to the skin flap and the dissection is carried superiorly, taking a segment of anterior rectus sheath along with the rectus muscle (see Fig. 10-10B). The deep inferior epigastric pedicle is divided and ligated. The rectus muscle should be divided superior to the arcuate line to minimize ventral weakness and subsequent herniation. The muscle is dissected

proximally to its origin along the lower medial costal cartilages. At least 1 cm of anterior rectus sheath should be preserved both medially and laterally to allow fascial closure. The superior epigastric vessels are identified and preserved. A suprafascial pocket is developed within the epigastric area to allow transfer of the myocutaneous flap to the mastectomy site. Care is taken to avoid torsion of the vascular pedicle.

Once the flap is transposed, it is tailored to fit the mastectomy defect (Fig. 10-10*B* and *C*). Some or all skin may be de-epithelialized to optimize contouring. The pectoral and rectus muscles are approximated, thus insetting the flap. Excess skin may be excised or buried to add projection or to fill the axillary defect but manipulation of the flap should be minimized to reduce the chances of flap necrosis. If necessary, subsequent contouring can be accomplished at the time of nipple reconstruction. Once symmetry has been optimized and the vascularity of the flap ensured, the dermis and skin are approximated (Fig. 10-10*D*). A closed-end drain is placed in the abdominal and mastectomy wounds and brought out through stab incisions in the pubic area and axilla, respectively.

Abdominal closure is completed by approximating the medial and lateral 1-cm rims of remaining rectus sheath. Polypropylene mesh may be used to reinforce the closure. The external oblique fascia can be mobilized and sutured to further strengthen the ventral wall.

The operative table is flexed to minimize tension on the abdominal closure. An abdominal binder is applied for support. Arm exercises and ambulation are begun at 48 to 96 hours, depending on the preference of the surgeon.

### COMPLICATIONS

Complications after RAM flap reconstruction have been evaluated and reported in several large series.[11-14] Major flap necrosis is infrequent, occurring in 0.3% to 3%. Conversely, small areas of fat necrosis may occur when the flap is harvested from the lower abdomen, where skin and fat outside of the territory of the deep superior epigastric vessels are encountered. The smoker or the morbidly obese (those having total body weight more than 100% of ideal body weight) have a higher than usual incidence of partial or major flap necrosis. Partial necrosis or small areas of fat necrosis are managed by resection, with primary or secondary closure.

Ventral hernias were common during the initial experience with RAM (0.3% to 8.3%),[11-14] some partly because attention was focused on ensuring optimal flap circulation in the early experience with this procedure. In so doing, the plastic surgeon left more anterior rectus sheath on the flap and less in the abdominal wall, making secure closure difficult and increasing the change of ventral weakness. Surgeons of the 1990s are adept in harvesting enough fascia to optimize RAM flap viability, while preserving adequate rectus fascia to prevent early as well as late ventral hernias or fascial weakness. After a 5-year follow-up on 137 pedicled RAM flaps, Mizgala and coworkers[13] in 1994 reported that 72% noted an improved abdominal appearance and 20% had improved posture. Forty-six percent experienced diminished abdominal strength, however, and 25% had a diminution in the ability to exercise; almost all of the patients have some hypoesthesia or dysesthesia of the skin of the abdominal wall. With bilateral rectus harvest, sit-up performance was slightly less than after unilateral transfer. Significant abdominal laxity to diffuse bulging without true hernia was noted in 11 of 150 patients. Six of these 11 patients gained an average of 11.7 lbs postoperatively. Mid-epigastric bulging occurred in 41%, compared with 6.1% of unoperated controls.

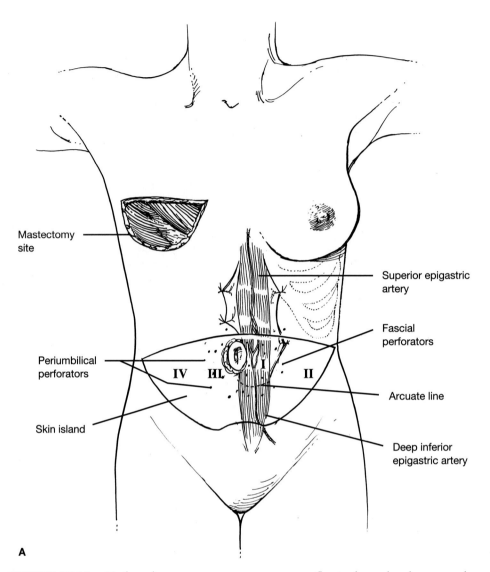

Mastectomy site

Superior epigastric artery

Fascial perforators

Periumbilical perforators

IV    III    I    II

Arcuate line

Skin island

Deep inferior epigastric artery

A

**FIGURE 10-10.** Unilateral transverse rectus myocutaneous flap is elevated and transposed to the chest, with resection of the less well-vascularized portions of the skin island. Portions of the flap are de-epithelialized and contoured. (**A**) Relationship of skin incisions to inferior epigastric vessels (fascial perforators). (**B**) Rotation of unilateral flap into position. (**C**) De-epithelialization of a portion of the flap. (**D**) Closure of incisions.

## *Double Rectus Abdominis Myocutaneous Flap Reconstruction*

### *INDICATIONS*

Patients undergoing bilateral mastectomies or a single mastectomy with sizable muscle and skin defects that cannot be covered using one rectus skin island may undergo bilateral rectus flap reconstruction. In situations in which radiation in-

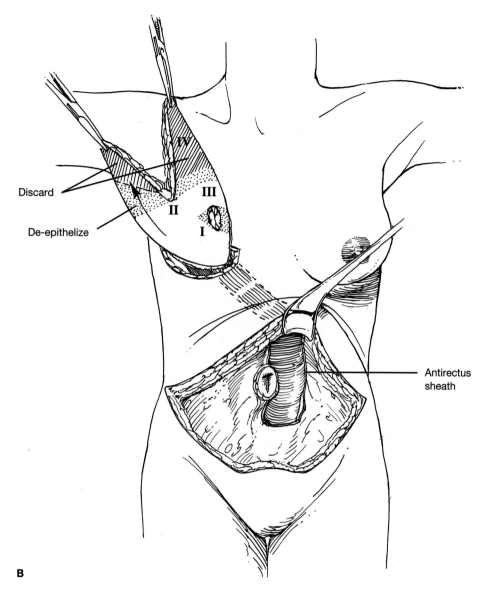

Discard

De-epithelize

Antirectus sheath

**B**

**FIGURE 10-10.** *(Continued)*

juries are extensive or resections of the osteocartilaginous chest wall are necessary, bilateral rectus flaps provide excellent coverage of defects, extending as high as the axilla.

## POSITIONING AND PREPARATION

Preparation extends from the clavicle to the mid-thigh and from posterior axillary line to posterior axillary line. Positioning is the same as for the unilateral rectus flap.

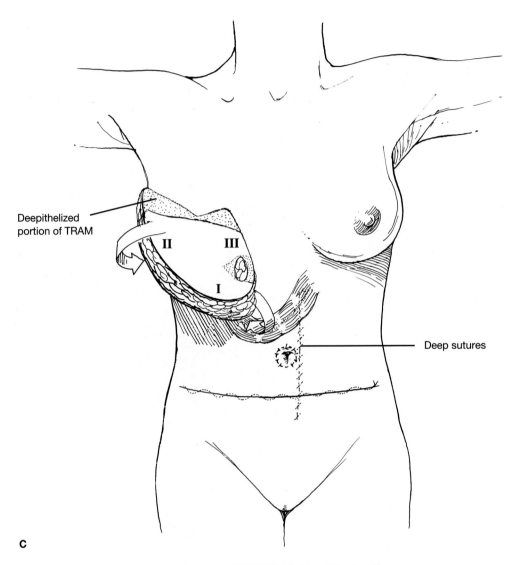

Deepithelized portion of TRAM

II    III

I

Deep sutures

**c**

**FIGURE 10-10.** *(Continued)*

### OPERATIVE PROCEDURE

A transverse skin island with a vertical component or bilateral vertical flaps can be designed as the defect requires. As noted previously, the vertical orientation is preferable in the morbidly obese patient. The amount of skin available with either a transverse or vertical skin island is greater with the use of both rectus muscles than in the unilateral procedure. The skin island is elevated to the lateral rectus sheath bilaterally. The sheath is incised on both sides, preserving at least 1 cm of medial and lateral anterior rectus sheath on each side and the linea alba. The rectus muscles are divided above the arcuate line, ligating the deep epigastric vessels, and are elevated in a cephalad direction to the costal margin, where the superior epigastric vessels are identified and preserved. If necessary, the lower costal margin can be resected to op-

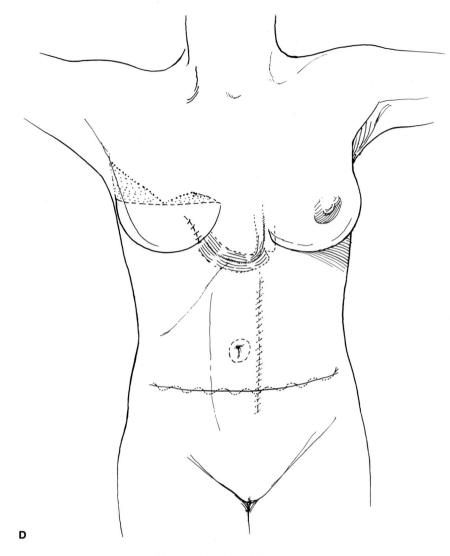

**D**

**FIGURE 10-10.** *(Continued)*

timize the arc of rotation. The flap is then transposed into the chest defect. If bilateral mastectomies have been performed, the skin to be transposed is incised in the midline, thus creating single flaps, which are transposed into the chest on each side. Submuscular implants or expanders are usually indicated after bilateral mastectomy. The postoperative course is similar to that after a single RAM flap. Progressive early ambulation is advised. A physical therapy program incorporating sit-ups and leg-raising exercises expedites recovery.

## COMPLICATIONS

The same risks apply as those noted with unilateral RAM flap transfer. Ventral weakness, hernia formation, or functional deficit are slightly more common after bilateral transfer. Given an intensive exercise program, most patients recover promptly and are able to resume normal daily functioning.

## Free-Flap Reconstruction of the Breast

### INDICATIONS

Free-tissue transfers from the lower abdomen, buttock, or lateral thigh are other options for reconstruction of the breast mound without use of implants. When the RAM flap is not available because of prior abdominal surgery or when it is not sufficiently large in the thin patient, a free flap can be used and can provide more tissue. Because the morbidity of a free flap is low, this procedure is often the first choice for reconstruction, especially when the plastic surgeon is well-versed in the technique. The well-vascularized free flap provides a generous amount of tissue for an aesthetic and natural-feeling breast, along with a hidden donor deformity. Complications of abdominal and back weakness associated with RAM reconstructions are minimized with free-tissue transfer of the rectus because less muscle is removed from its normal position and more tissue is provided to the chest area.

Potential sources of myocutaneous free flaps are (1) the lower abdomen, based on the deep inferior epigastric vessels; (2) the superior and inferior gluteal, based on each respective artery; and (3) the lateral thigh flap, using lateral femoral vessels.

### POSITIONING, PREPARATION, AND OPERATIVE TECHNIQUE

The patient is placed in the prone or lateral decubitus position for harvesting either gluteal (Fig. 10-11A and B) or lateral thigh flaps. The supine position is used for the lower abdominal free flap (Fig. 10-12). Once the skin island is outlined, a segment of muscle along with the vascular pedicle is isolated and divided. The fascia and cutaneous defects are closed. The patient is then positioned in the supine position. Using the operating microscope, arterial and venous repairs are performed to revascularize the tissue transfer. The internal mammary, thoracoacromial, thoracodorsal, axillary, or cephalic vessels can be used for repair. A light dressing is applied. Subsequently, bra support increases comfort and may aid healing and contouring of the breast mound.

### COMPLICATIONS

The most significant concern after this type of surgery is arterial or venous thrombosis of the microvascular repairs. Technical difficulties in performing microvascular repairs or prolonged ischemia time may contribute to thrombosis of the microscopic anastomoses, resulting in partial or total loss of the flap. Some surgeons, therefore, prefer to perform this as a separate procedure. At UCLA and many centers across the country, immediate free-flap reconstruction has become a preferred approach, which can often be completed in 3 to 6 hours, although when bilateral gluteal reconstructions are necessary, 6 or more hours can be added to the procedure. Hematoma and infection are relatively infrequent but may occur at the donor site or at the chest wall recipient site.

The small amount of muscle harvested with these flaps rarely leads to functional deficit at the donor site. The incidence of dysesthesia and weakness of the abdominal wall is lower after the free rectus flap than after RAM. Patients only infrequently develop difficulty in ambulating after gluteal free flaps. Physical therapy usually yields quick resolution of any temporary disability. Lengthy preoperative discussions are crucial to ensure that patients understand the personal ramifications of microvascular reconstructive efforts. In experienced hands, patients do well and are exceptionally pleased with the aesthetic outcome.

## Nipple–Areola Reconstruction

The breast mound undergoes dynamic changes during the first 3 months after reconstruction, regardless of the form of reconstruction. For this reason, nipple–areola reconstructions are usually performed no sooner than 3 months after recreation of the breast mound. Many patients may choose not to undergo nipple reconstruction because the reconstructed breast mound provides suitable symmetry in clothing. Nipple reconstruction is a relatively simple procedure, however, which can be completed in a 30- to 60-minute outpatient procedure under local anesthesia.

### SURGICAL OPTIONS

The key to reconstruction of the areola is to match the skin color of the contralateral areola. By harvesting full-thickness skin grafts from various areas of the body, a color similar to the contralateral side can usually be obtained. Possible donor sites include supraclavicular or postauricular areas for pale areolar skin; groin crease or medial thigh for pink skin; or gluteal fold, inner thigh, or labia for dark brown or even highly pigmented skin.

There are numerous forms of nipple reconstruction, including nipple-sharing, earlobe graft, ear cartilage graft, fat grafts, and toe pulp. A skate technique that effectively reproduces and retains nipple prominence has been described. A modification of the skate technique is illustrated in Figure 10-13A through F.[15] Atrophy is far less common with this form of reconstruction. Patient and surgeon satisfaction has been high.

### OPERATIVE TECHNIQUE

A symmetric position is determined preoperatively with the patient in the standing position. A skin–fat flap (modified skate) is elevated to create a new nipple. After nipple reconstruction, the graft is harvested and sutured into position (Fig. 10-14A through E). Tattooing can be used to simulate the areola at the time of nipple reconstruction or tattooing can be used to match the contralateral areolar skin color (Fig. 10-15).

### COMPLICATIONS

Loss of nipple height of about 3 to 5 mm can occur with the skate technique. This loss of height should be anticipated in planning the height and dimension of the nipple. Partial or complete sloughing of the areolar graft may be due to

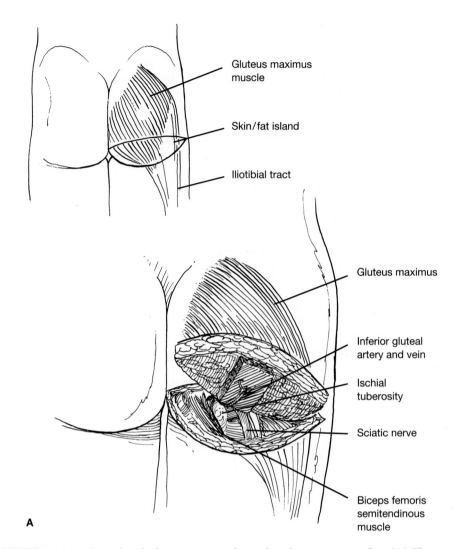

Gluteus maximus muscle

Skin/fat island

Iliotibial tract

Gluteus maximus

Inferior gluteal artery and vein

Ischial tuberosity

Sciatic nerve

Biceps femoris semitendinous muscle

A

**FIGURE 10-11.** Procedure for harvesting an inferior gluteal myocutaneous flap. (**A**) The patient is turned supine after harvest of the flap with the patient in the prone position. Microvascular anastomosis is then accomplished. (**B**) The donor defect is illustrated.

subgraft hematoma or mobility. Use of a compression dressing usually avoids both complications. When graft sloughing has occurred, nipple tattooing may be effective in centering the areola and in improving color match with the contralateral areola.

## *Breast Reconstruction After Partial Mastectomy and Radiation*

Reconstruction after a partial mastectomy and radiation therapy raises several important questions:

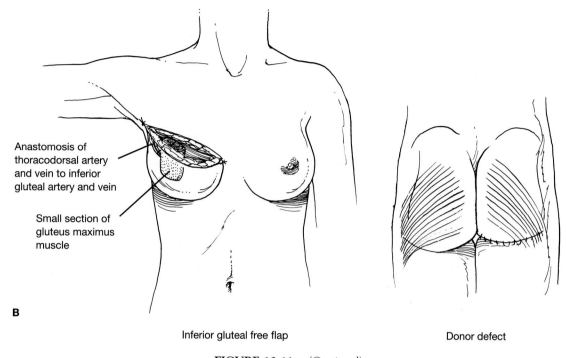

Anastomosis of
thoracodorsal artery
and vein to inferior
gluteal artery and vein

Small section of
gluteus maximus
muscle

B

Inferior gluteal free flap                    Donor defect

**FIGURE 10-11.** *(Continued)*

When is reconstruction required?

What is the ideal management for the common signs and symptoms?

What are the strategies for cancer treatment and subsequent reconstruction?

What is the role of implants after radiation therapy?

## REASONS FOR RECONSTRUCTION

In a 10-year retrospective review of 807 breast cancers treated by partial mastectomy and radiation at the University of Massachusetts Medical Center (personal communication, E. Matory, 1995), 46 patients presented for evaluation and treatment of postradiation deformity: recurrent cancer, 19; ulceration–infection, 3; breast deformity, 15; firmness, 3; pain, 1; volume deficit, 4; retraction, 4; nipple displacement, 3. These problems and their potential therapeutic solutions can be classified as follows:

    I.   Salvage mastectomy for recurrent cancer, ulceration, or infection

   II.   Dissatisfied patients complaining of breast pain, firmness, and nipple or breast retraction or both

 III.   Dissatisfaction because of breast asymmetry or volume deficit

       A.   Breasts that were soft, supple, with minimal ptosis, with adequate but not excessive remaining breast

       B.   Overall breast volume was severely ptotic or more than 100 g

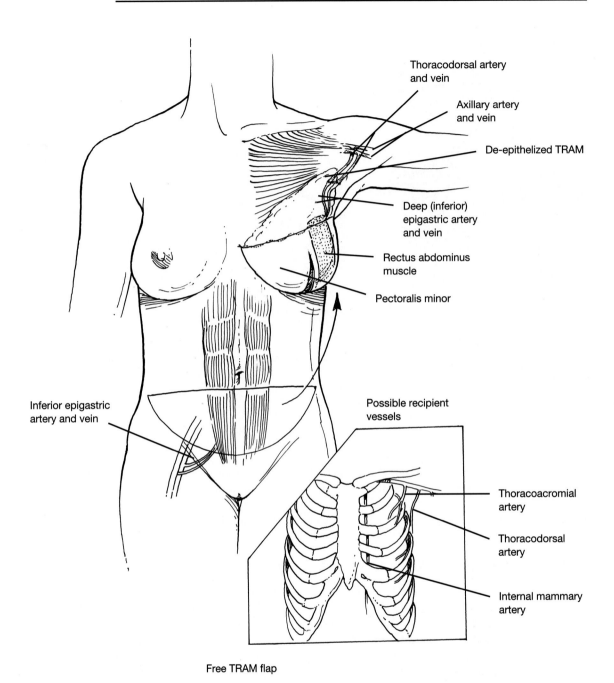

Thoracodorsal artery and vein

Axillary artery and vein

De-epithelized TRAM

Deep (inferior) epigastric artery and vein

Rectus abdominus muscle

Pectoralis minor

Inferior epigastric artery and vein

Possible recipient vessels

Thoracoacromial artery

Thoracodorsal artery

Internal mammary artery

Free TRAM flap

**FIGURE 10-12.** The transverse rectus myocutaneous flap can be transferred to the chest, with a microscopic anastomosis between the inferior epigastric vessels and those in the chest wall.

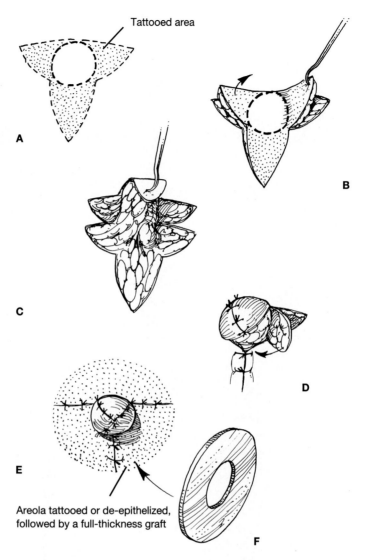

Tattooed area

A

B

C

D

E

Areola tattooed or de-epithelized,
followed by a full-thickness graft

F

**FIGURE 10-13.** De-epithelialized skin and fat are manipulated to form a new nipple.

### IDEAL MANAGEMENT

Ionizing radiation causes acute and chronic changes to all tissues within an irradiated field. Inability of cells to replicate, often accompanied by cell death, commonly results in poor healing after traumatic, surgical, or infectious injury. Because of the severe devascularization and wound healing difficulties of the irradiated bed, additional blood supply is required to treat these patients. Immediate autologous chest wall reconstruction or immediate autologous breast reconstruction may be accomplished with a latissimus dorsi myocutaneous, pedicled, or microvascular TRAM or with microvascular gluteal flap alternatives. Reconstructions for nonlife-threatening or mild to moderate deformities should not be undertaken before 1 year from initial therapy to allow maximal resolution of the acute inflammatory processes.

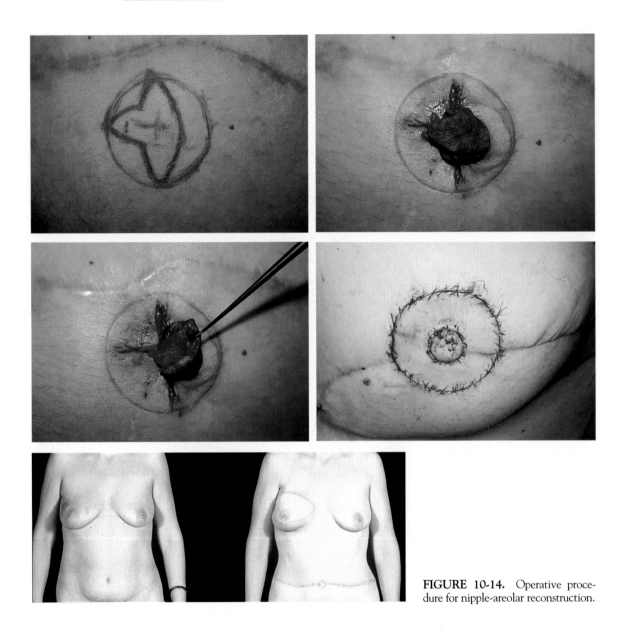

**FIGURE 10-14.** Operative procedure for nipple-areolar reconstruction.

## *ROLE OF IMPLANTS AFTER RADIATION THERAPY*

Any nonvascularized reconstruction such as an implant must have overlying tissues with excellent blood supply. Radiation inflicts injury to the DNA contained in all cells of living tissues in the irradiated zone. The resultant endovascular injury affects skin, ribs, residual breast, muscle, lung, and heart. The acute injury phase, lasting 6 weeks, may be associated with erythema, pain, and edema. The chronic phase is characterized by fibrosis, atrophy, telangiectasis, and poor wound healing. Undermining these devascularized tissues to place an implant is rarely without complication. For that reason, when augmentation is desired, it should be accomplished with some type of autologous flap.

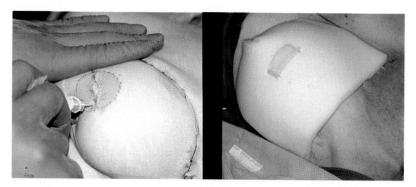

**FIGURE 10-15.** Tattooing to simulate areola at time of nipple reconstruction.

## REFERENCES

1. Snyderman RK, Guthrie RH. Reconstruction of the female breast afterave radical mastectomy. Plast Reconstr Surg 1971;47:565.
2. Gruber RP, Khan RA, Lash H, et al. Breast reconstruction following mastectomy: a comparison of submuscular and subcutaneous techniques. Plast Reconstr Surg 1981;67:312.
3. Goldwyn RM. Breast reconstruction after mastectomy. N Engl J Med 1987;317:1711.
4. Asplund O. Capsular contracture in silicone gel and saline-filled breast implants after reconstruction. Plast Reconstr Surg 1984;73:270.
5. Gylbert L, Asplung O, Jurell G. Capsular contracture after breast reconstruction with silicone-gel and saline-filled implants: a 6-year follow-up. Plast Reconstr Surg 1990;85:373.
6. Radovan C. Breast reconstruction after mastectomy using a temporary expander. Plast Reconstr Surg 1982;69:195.
7. Gibney J. The long-term results of tissue expansion for breast reconstruction. Clin Plast Surg 1987;14:509.
8. Becker H. The permanent tissue expander. Clin Plast Surg 1987;14:519.
9. Argenta LC, Marks MW, Grabb WC. Selective use of serial expansion in breast reconstruction. Ann Plast Surg 1983;11:188.
10. Versaci AD. Reconstruction of a pendulous breast utilizing a tissue expander. Clin Plast Surg 1987;14(3):499.
11. McCraw JB, Horton CE, Grossman JA, et al. An early appraisal of the methods of tissue expansion and the transverse rectus abdomins musculocutaneous flap in reconstruction of the breast following mastectomy. Ann Plast Surg 1987;18:93.
12. Hartrampf CR Jr. The transverse abdominal island flap for breast reconstruction. A 7-year experience. Clin Plast Surg 1988;15:703.
13. Mizgala C, Hartrampf CR Jr, Bennett K. Assessment of abdominal wall surgery after pedicled TRAM flap surgery: 5 to 7 year follow-up of 150 consecutive patients. Plast Recontr Surg 1994;93:988.
14. Hartrampf CR Jr. Abdominal wall competence in transverse abdominal island flap operation. Ann Plast Surg 1984;12:139.
15. Spear SL. A modified skate flap for nipple-areolar reconstruction. Presented at the Annual Meeting of the American Society of Plastic and Reconstructive Surgeons, Seattle, 1991.

# Part

# V

## Technical Approaches for the Treatment of Common Benign Disorders

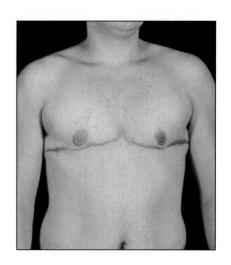

*Atlas of Techniques in Breast Surgery,*
by William Silen, W. Earle Matory, Jr. and Susan M. Love.
Lippincott-Raven Publishers, Philadelphia, © 1996.

# *Chapter* 11

# Procedures for Addressing Benign Disease

## ✦ *MICRODOCHECTOMY*

### *Indications*

A spontaneous unilateral bloody or serous nipple discharge that emanates from one duct requires definitive diagnosis. Discharge may be grossly bloody, or sticky and clear and positive for occult blood. The only instance in which grossly bloody discharge is encountered in the absence of a pathologic lesion is during the terminal stages of pregnancy, in which case the discharge invariably disappears spontaneously after delivery.

### *Surgical Planning, Localization*

Identifying a trigger zone by palpation is often useful but may be misleading. We find preoperative ductogram to be a helpful diagnostic tool, serving a dual purpose. Ductograms may establish the nature of the pathology; more importantly, the site of intraductal pathology can often be defined. Although most intraductal papillomas lie adjacent to the areola, other sources of gross or occult bloody discharge do not. Intraductal carcinoma in situ, for example, may be located more distally along the duct and can be easily missed if only a small portion of a major duct adjacent to the nipple is removed. In addition, the duct sometimes takes unusual twists and turns, which are difficult to anticipate preoperatively. A good ductogram helps to clarify ductal anatomy. Smears of nipple discharge to search for malignant cells are not usually diagnostic because false-positive and false-negative results are frequently encountered.

145

Sartorius and Smith have recommended a technique for preoperative localization of the duct in question.[1] The distance of the lesion from the nipple is measured on the ductogram and a piece of 0 polypropylene (Prolene) is cut to the same length. This is threaded into the duct, knotted at the most proximal end, and kept in place with a drop of collodion. The polypropylene blue suture is easily visible within the duct during dissection and serves as a marker of the extent of excision necessary to remove the tumor.

Another preoperative marking technique can be used when the tumor is close to the nipple and completely obstructs the duct. Methylene blue dye is instilled into the discharging duct preoperatively and sealed in the duct with collodion. The dye identifies the duct and the site of resection. When the intraductal lesion is demonstrated on ductogram to be 1 cm or more from the nipple, we have found that wire localization helps to identify the lesion and limits the extent of the dissection for diagnosis and treatment. This is particularly true in lesions of the smaller branches of the duct.

If the tumor is at or adjacent to the nipple, a circumareolar incision is made under local anesthesia and dissected medially toward the involved duct (Fig. 11-1). At the nipple, the duct is identified by the suture, dye, or blood within the duct (see Fig. 11-1). Just at the underside of the nipple, a small mosquito clamp is passed around the duct, and the most proximal tip of the duct is ligated. The clamp remains on the distal end for retraction. The duct is carefully dissected distally for the distance determined by the suture, dye, or preoperative ductogram. Once the lesion has been reached, the distal end of the duct is doubly ligated and excised. A small amount of breast parenchyma is excised with the involved duct. When the dissection is completed, the fibrous tissue within the subareolar area can be used to accomplish a layered closure. The wound is closed with 3-0 polydioxone (Vicryl) intradermally, followed by 4-0 polyioxanone (PDS) or monofilament polyglyconate (Maxon). If the tumor is far removed from the nipple and requires needle localization, the operative procedure is identical to that described in Chapter 4.

## Complications

Failure to remove the offending lesion is more common than generally recognized. Sometimes an incorrect diagnosis of ductal ectasia is given, when actually a dilated duct has been removed, without excision of the obstructing lesion. Under these circumstances, nipple discharge ceases but the lesion remains untreated. Preoperative ductogram is helpful in avoiding this pitfall.

Nipple or areolar distortion may occur as a result of excessive undermining of the areola. Retraction of parenchyma beneath the areola contributes to nipple–areolar disfigurement. Preoperative localization of these tumors minimizes the extent of dissection and postoperative nipple–areolar distortion.

## ✦ CHRONIC SUBAREOLAR ABSCESSES AND FISTULAS

Chronic subareolar abscesses are particularly difficult to treat. A common initial manifestation is that of an acute abscess adjacent to the nipple. The original lesion is easily incised and drained, and the wound is allowed to heal secondarily. Even

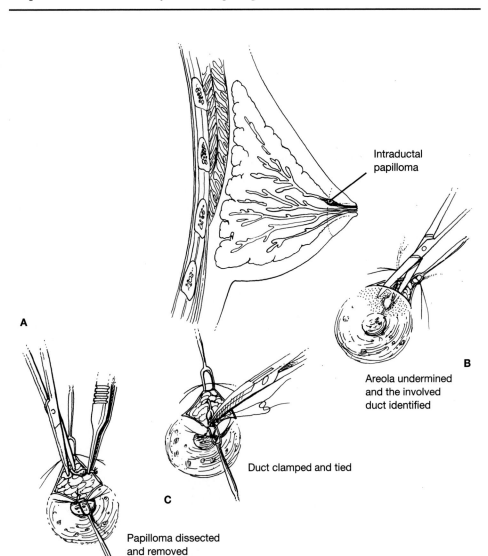

Intraductal
papilloma

A

B

Areola undermined
and the involved
duct identified

Duct clamped and tied

C

Papilloma dissected
and removed

D

Microdochectomy

**FIGURE 11-1.** Microdochectomy.

though the acute inflammation resolves, abscesses often recur, with periodic exacerbations and remissions.

The key to permanent resolution is an understanding of the pathophysiology of the chronic subareolar abscess. Classic teaching purports that a blocked mammary duct becomes secondarily infected with a resultant abscess that forms along the areolar border. Although this presumed etiology may be present in some cases, true ductal obstruction is most commonly identified during lactation and has an entirely different course. In this situation, milk stagnates in the periphery of the breast, resulting in a swollen wedge or phlegmon of breast tissue. Secondary infection may or may not supervene but when it does, the resultant abscess is rarely near or immediately adjacent to the areola.

Updated reviews of nipple architecture suggest the possibility of a different cause of chronic subareolar abscess. Attempts to cannulate breast ducts at the nipple have shown that there are many "blind ducts" that extend for only 1 to 2 cm, without connection to breast parenchyma (Fig. 11-2). These orifices most likely represent sebaceous glands, which secrete a fine waxy material that coats the nipple and prevents irritation during breast-feeding. Many authorities believe that chronic subareolar abscess is caused by infection of one of these blind sebaceous glands, with progression to a subareolar abscess. Pathologic analysis of these lesions commonly identifies granulation tissue and squamous metaplasia consistent with this proposed pathogenesis. There are instances in which true ductal ectasia is present in virtually all or most of the true major mammary ducts, in association with breeches in ductal epithelial integrity and sub-

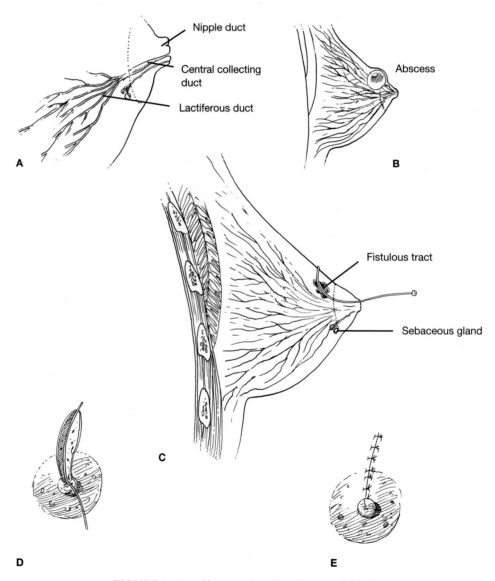

**FIGURE 11-2.**  Chronic subareolar abscess and fistula.

sequent chronic inflammation in the breast tissue itself (plasma cell mastitis). These should be distinguished if possible from recurrent infections of the areolar sebaceous glands and from hidradenitis suppurativa. True mammary duct ectasia responds well to excision of all of the major ducts through a circumareolar incision.

As with glandular infections in other parts of the body, one must remove the entire affected modified sebaceous gland to prevent recurrence when an infected sebaceous gland is the cause of the problem. Definitive treatment of these chronic infections is best addressed when they are quiescent. The presence of tenderness, fever, erythema, and pain indicates acute inflammation and significant bacteriologic contamination that will likely cause infection of the operative wound. These chronically inflamed areas are difficult to anesthetize solely with local anesthesia. The addition of short-acting general anesthetic agents such as propofol enable a more comfortable and more definitive procedure. Perioperative antibiotics are deemed beneficial. Note that recurrent chronic abscesses are usually the result of inadequate removal of involved ducts or glands or resections in the presence of severe bacterial contamination.

### Operative Technique

After the patient has been prepared and draped, the tract of gland should be cannulated, usually with a Prolene suture.

A radial incision incorporating the duct orifice in the nipple is preferable because it facilitates complete removal of the offending sebaceous gland. Although a circumareolar incision affords a better cosmetic result, it may not allow complete removal of an infected sebaceous gland. When a circumareolar incision is used for an infected sebaceous gland, the opening at the areolar margin should be cored out and the tract followed to the nipple.

The incision is outlined with a marking pencil to include the designated ductal orifices in a small radial elliptical incision (see Fig. 11-2*D*). Electrocautery is used to dissect and excise the entire tract. Hemostasis is confirmed, and the wound is irrigated with an antibiotic solution. We suggest avoiding primary wound closure. Allow the cavity to heal by secondary intent, or use a delayed primary closure in 3 to 5 days. Antibiotics are continued for about 7 days. Wounds that are left open may compromise the cosmetic outcome but the incidence of acute or chronic postoperative infection is less.

### Complications

In the best of hands, the incidence of recurrence ranges from 10% to 50%. Repeat infections may necessitate multiple deforming procedures, often accompanied by a debilitating postoperative course. The final resolution may require resection of the nipple-areolor complex but does not require masectomy.

## ✦ BREAST MASSES IN THE PUBESCENT FEMALE

Breast development is inhibited or severely compromised if the nipple bud is excised in the pubescent female. Breast cancer is rare in this age group and watchful waiting is generally recommended for breast masses in this stage of life. Lymphomas and cystosarcoides phyllodes occur occasionally, however. Fine-needle aspiration biopsy can be performed with minimal risk to breast development.

## ✦ ACCESSORY BREAST PARENCHYMA, NIPPLES

The most common location of accessory breast parenchyma is the axilla. The breast mound is situated in a subcutaneous plane and can usually be removed entirely without entering the axillary or pectoral fascia. Carcinomas occasionally develop in accessory breast tissue in the axilla. An accessory nipple–areola without an associated glandular component can be excised as an ellipse.

## ✦ GYNECOMASTIA

Gynecomastia, male breast enlargement, is the result of an increase in fibrofatty or mammary tissue. The relative increase in each of these tissues varies from one patient to another. A wide variety of drugs are associated with the development of gynecomastia. Steroids (ingested by body builders), diuretics, antiepileptics, cholesterol-lowering drugs, $H_2$-blockers (cimetidine), and many other agents have been implicated.[2] Of note, idiopathic gynecomastia or even instances secondary to medications may be unilateral. In most instances, the diagnosis of gynecomastia is easily established by simple physical examination, which demonstrates a typical relatively firm smooth button of breast tissue about 2 cm in diameter immediately deep to the areola and nipple. A variable increase in surrounding dense adipose tissue is noted. Biopsy is unnecessary in a patient who is taking one of the above drugs and who has the characteristic examination. Should there be any doubt regarding the true nature of the lesion, biopsy is indicated.

Adolescent gynecomastia is commonly transient. Any contemplated operation should be deferred until near completion of sexual maturity, as defined by secondary sexual development (pubic, scrotal, and axillary hair, muscular and skeletal growth). Psychosocial ramifications of gynecomastia almost uniformly lead to some degree of social isolation, depression, and a lack of self-esteem. These symptoms are often of significant magnitude, so that the adolescent and the adult are likely to reap considerable emotional benefit from surgical reduction of the gynecomastia.

### *Anatomic Considerations*

The anatomic and aesthetic characteristics of the male breast are not widely recognized. When supine, the normal male areola is positioned at the level of or within 1 cm of the lateral pectoral border, just lateral to the mid-clavicular line. When sitting, the areola is 2 to 3 cm below this position. There are variable thicknesses and contours within the male breast, as is the case in the female. The thickness of skin and adipose tissue is greatest inferior to the pectoral border and is thinner (1 cm) in most remaining areas. Subareolar thickness should contribute to no more than 4 mm of areolar projection above the surrounding skin. Subareolar prominence may be as much as 1 to 2 cm if there is considerable underlying pectoral hypertrophy. A hypertrophied pectoral muscle makes the entire chest prominent, particularly in the subareolar area. An overly large resection of breast tissue and fat results in an unattractive central depression, which is difficult to repair. If the pectoral muscles are thick, subareolar fullness must be maintained to preserve symmetry and avoid deformity.

Skin redundancy often accompanies gynecomastia, especially in the large-breasted patient. In the past, excessive skin was excised, often leading to widened scars and dysesthesia. Fibrofatty reduction with suction lipectomy, followed by subareolar glandular excision through a circumareolar approach, minimizes the extent of dissection and makes contouring of the breast simpler and less extensive than direct excision. As a result of the reduced adipose and glandular volume, the skin envelope retracts with time, eliminating the need for skin resection. If some excess skin persists after 6 months, the typically smaller cutaneous resection can be performed as a secondary outpatient procedure.

## Operative Techniques

The distribution of breast fullness is assessed in the supine and upright positions and outlined on the skin. The anticipated reduction of the subareolar and medial breast is usually less than that within the lateral and infra-areolar areas or that within the axillary tail. This variable fat distribution is best delineated preoperatively using skin markings. The distribution of fat may change in the supine position, and adjustments in the amount of resection or suction aspiration should be made accordingly to achieve the relative thicknesses of fat that contribute to an aesthetic male-pattern breast contour.

Aspiration of fat from prominent areas of the breast is facilitated by the injection of a large volume (400 to 750 mL) of fluid into the tissues. This is accomplished by using a dilute solution (usually about 0.25%) Xylocaine to stay well within the nontoxic dose (less than 5 mg/kg). The injected fluid is aspirated during the procedure. Cannulas of 3 to 4 mm in diameter are used to reduce all but 2 cm thickness of subcutaneous fat in the lower breast and 1 cm elsewhere, thus yielding a more masculine contour. Once aspiration is complete, a small subareolar glandular core remains. This is reduced through a circumareolar incision, which is placed about 1 mm within the areola–cutaneous junction to minimize visibility of the scar.

The nipple–areolar skin, along with 1 to 2 cm of subcutaneous fat, is elevated from the underlying parenchyma. The subareolar core is grasped with Allis clamps and resected along a suprafascial plane. The resected specimen is sent to pathology, along with the aspirated fat. Hemostasis is confirmed. Closed suction drains, if deemed appropriate, are brought out through axillary stab incisions to assist closure of the resultant dead space. The retained layer of subcutaneous fat hides areas of depression or irregularity of contour.

## Complications

Hematomas and seromas are common after reduction of a gynecomastia. The vigorous activity of the male gender may contribute to these complications. Large skin–fat flaps should be drained to allow a fibrin seal between the subcutaneous fat and the chest wall. Additional visible scarring is minimized by using a drain site in the hair-

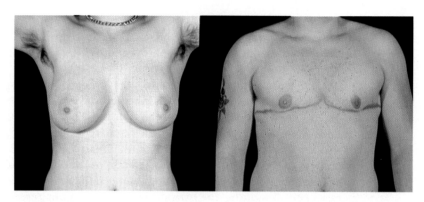

**FIGURE 11-3.** Before and after treatment of gynecomastia. Excellent result.

bearing axilla. Visible circumareolar scarring is unusual when the incision for parenchymal reduction is placed just within the areolar–cutaneous junction. Areolar distortions may occur if the preoperative skin alignment is not maintained. To minimize soft-tissue trauma, forceful retraction of the skin edges during surgery should be avoided. Hypertrophy of the cutaneous scar is common but approximation with slowly resorbed sutures may minimize hypertrophy. Deep dermal PDS or Maxon with a running intradermal polypropylene (Prolene) suture left in for an extended period, 6 to 8 weeks, is effective.

The patient should be made fully aware of the possibility of postoperative asymmetry before operation. Analysis of preoperative photographs helps the patient to see and understand preoperative asymmetry and enhances the surgeon's identification and subsequent management of differences in contour and appearance of the nipple. Postoperative irregularity can be minimized by a clear understanding of the ideal male breast contours and relation to male anatomy (Fig. 11-3). In the best of hands, however, depressions or irregularities may be noted intra- and postoperatively. Primary or secondary suction contouring or autologous fat injection are usually effective solutions.

Loss of nipple and breast sensation, common after a surgical resection of a gynecomastia, is rare after aspiration reduction alone. If this complication occurs after the latter, it is temporary and usually resolves within 3 to 6 months.

### REFERENCES

1. Sartorius OWS, Smith HS. Contract ductography for the recognition and localization of benign and malignant breast lesions: an improved technique. In: Logan W, ed. Breast Carcinoma. New York: Wiley, 1977.
2. Braunstein GD. Gynecomastia. N Engl J Med 1993;328:490.

*Atlas of Techniques in Breast Surgery,*
by William Silen, W. Earle Matory, Jr. and Susan M. Love.
Lippincott-Raven Publishers, Philadelphia, © 1996.

# *Index*

*Note:* Page numbers followed by *f* indicate figures; those followed by *t* indicate tables.